Know Your Sweets

A Basic Guide on the Different Sugar Substitutes and Sweeteners

MARY CONRAD

ISBN: 1548244856
ISBN-13: 978-1548244859

DEDICATION

This book is for my Mom, who was lost to cancer but fought bravely for three years. Love you, Mom!

MARY CONRAD

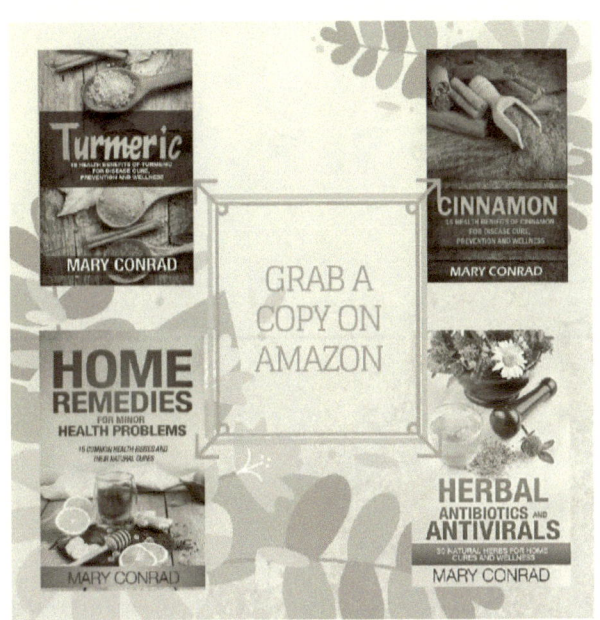

Disclaimer

This book provides general information, personal experiences and extensive research regarding health and related subjects. The information provided in this book, and in any linked materials, is based on my own personal experience and is for informational purposes only. It is not intended to be interpreted as a professional medical advice. Speak with your physician or a trusted healthcare professional prior to taking any nutritional or herbal supplements. Please keep in mind that reactions and results may vary from each individual due to differences in state of health

Before considering any guidance from this book, please ensure you do not have any underlying health conditions, which may interfere with the suggested healing methods. If the reader or any other person has a medical concern or pre-existing condition, please consult with an appropriately licensed physician or healthcare professional. Never disregard professional medical advice or delay in seeking it because of something you have read in this book or in any linked materials.

Table of Contents

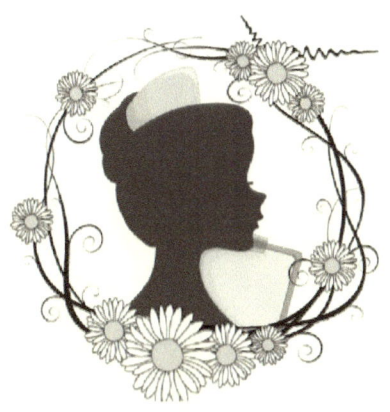

Introduction

Sugar is one of the most decadent creations to grace the human palate. It's hard to deny that eating sweet desserts and adding sweeteners to drinks and beverages add to the whole heavenly experience. Although it's sweet, sugar can be both addictive and detrimental to health when abused. For those with conditions such as diabetes, controlling calories and sugar intake becomes a way of life.

With the predominance of the use of sugar from drinks, processed food and baked goods, knowledge is essential to get a better idea on whether the type of sugar used is suited to both taste and health goals. This book provides a concise overview of regular sugar, which sets the stage for a discussion about the different types of sugar substitutes. When people talk about sugar, they usually refer to the most common type, table sugar. But there are many alternatives to refined sugar. There are natural and artificial sugar substitutes, as well as modified sugars and sugar alcohols.

In reality, sugar is more complicated than just the white powdery stuff on the counter or the light-yellow syrup inside a bottle. Using the right one and avoiding the unhealthy ones can make a difference to both health and wellness. Read on, try the different types of sugar, and may you find something that suits your sweet palate and may benefit your health.

MARY CONRAD

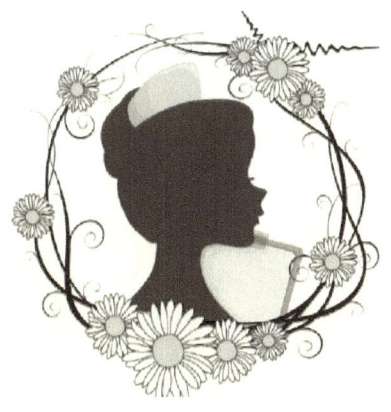

Chapter 1

Overview of Regular Sugar

A book about sugar substitutes is not complete without at least an overview of what they are substituting: original or regular sugar. This chapter provides a rundown of the origins, types, and benefits of sugar in general. This sets the stage for a more thorough discussion of sugar substitutes in the succeeding chapters. It puts sugar substitutes in perspective, and allows for a deeper appreciation and understanding of these different types of sweeteners.

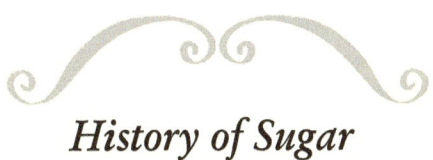

History of Sugar

Sugar is a sweet and soluble form of carbohydrates. When people talk about sugar, they most often refer to table/granulated sugar. As

1

its name suggests, it is the type of sugar that is usually served in tables, whether in households or in restaurants. It is the regular or default sugar manufactured from sugarcane or sugar beets.

In the ancient times, the only sweetener available was honey. Sugar as we know it today is believed to have originated from Polynesia, spreading to India where the method of crystallization was developed, then to Persia (Iran), Africa, Europe, New World (America), and the rest of the world. Colonization, religious crusades, and trade routes served as vehicles for bringing sugar all over the globe.

Natural philosopher Gaius Plinius Secundus, also known as Pliny the Elder, described sugar in his encyclopedia *Natural History*: *"It is a kind of honey found in cane, white as gum, and it crunches between the teeth. It comes in lumps the size of a hazelnut. Sugar is used only for medical purposes."*

How far sugar has come! While sugar is still used for medical purposes notably in the form of dextrose which serves as food for hospitalized folks, sugar is more popular for its role in the daily lives of people as an ingredient that makes food and beverages sweet.

Types of Sugar

There are 3 types of sugar based on the type or number of compounds. Let us break down the sweet stuff.

Monosaccharides

These are simple sugars. There are 3 sub-types.

> ➢ **Glucose** is dextrose or grape sugar. It is naturally found in fruits and plant juices, hence a primary product of photosynthesis. It is also known as "blood sugar" because it

is the simplest unit of sugar that directly enters the bloodstream. Hence, dextrose is given to patients who are bedridden, newly-operated, or in conditions wherein they do not have the capacity to consume food orally.

- ➤ **Fructose** is fruit sugar or levulose. It naturally occurs in fruits and some root vegetables. It is the sweetest of sugars.

- ➤ **Galactose** is a component of milk sugar. It does not occur by itself but with glucose to form lactose. It is less sweet than glucose.

Disaccharides

These are compound sugars, formed by combining 2 monosaccharides by hydrolysis or by taking away a molecule of water. There are also 3 sub-types.

- ➤ **Sucrose** is what we know as regular sugar, table sugar, or granulated sugar. Sucrose is hydrolized sugarcane or sugar beet. It is made by combining glucose and fructose via hydrolysis.

- ➤ **Maltose** is malt sugar. It comes from malted grain, from barley to malt. It is made by combining glucose and another glucose.

- ➤ **Lactose** is milk sugar. It is a combination of galactose and glucose. It is digested by the body via the enzyme lactase. Babies have this enzyme, allowing them to digest breast milk. However, some adults lack or do not have this enzyme, making them lactose intolerant or lactase deficient.

Oligosaccharides or Polysaccharides

These have longer chains of sugars. Technically, they have 2 or more monosaccharides. Examples are human breast milk, starch, soybeans, and fiber-rich plants such as artichoke, asparagus, onions, leeks, chicory, and burdock.

These are the types and sub-types of sugar. There are other chemicals that are sweet but not sugar, such as glycerol.

Types of Sucrose or Regular Sugar

There are several types of sucrose or regular sugar.

Granulated Sugar is also called refined, table, or white sugar. It is highly-refined, multi-purpose, and not prone to caking.

Caster Sugar is the finest of granulated white sugar used in baking and beverages. It is also called superfine, ultrafine, or bar.

Powdered Sugar is known as confectioners or icing sugar, made by adding cornstarch to finely-ground white sugar to prevent caking. It is often used in icing and dusting.

Decorative Sugars are coarse or large granules of sugar used for decorating confections. There are two types: pearl sugar and sanding sugar.

Brown Sugar is white sugar with molasses added back. It tastes earthy and caramel-like, and has a moist and sandy texture. It can be light or dark, depending on the amount of molasses added.

Muscovado/Barbados Sugar (UK), *Turbinado Sugar* (US), and *Demerara Sugar* (UK) are partially-processed raw sugar. This means that the molasses is not removed, resulting to a sticky and grainy texture with strong and rich flavor. They look like brown sugar.

These types of sugars can come in various forms: granulated, liquid/syrup, or cubes.

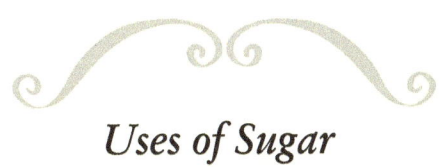

Uses of Sugar

Sugar enhances the taste and texture of food and drinks, specifically the palatability of nutrient-rich food. It balances saltiness, sourness, bitterness, spiciness, and acidity. It is used to sweeten drinks, food, and baked goods. In baking, sugar can form a brown crust – a process known as Maillard reaction. It is also used as a preservative to make jams, marmalades, preserves, and candied treats. In manufacturing, its byproducts serve as components of fuel.

The *2015-2020 Dietary Guidelines for Americans* summarized the benefits of sugar: *"Added sugars provide sweetness that can help improve the palatability of foods, help with preservation, and/or contribute to functional attributes such as viscosity, texture, body, color, and browning capability."*

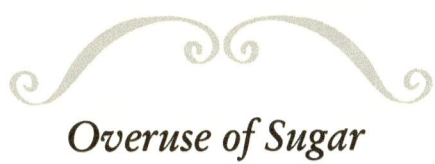

Overuse of Sugar

Fat used to be a health culprit, but recent years shifted the blame to sugar. Studies show that excessive intake of sugar can lead to a gamut of health conditions including diabetes, tooth decay, hyperactivity, obesity, cardiovascular disease, metabolic dysfunction, inflammation, dementia, and macular degeneration. Experimental studies are inconclusive, but anecdotal claims point to the need to regulate sugar intake.

While sugar is essentially a necessary macronutrient and can satisfy one's sweet tooth, too much of it, like any other food or nutrient, is bad for the body. It is especially dangerous when it comes in the form of empty calories, notably in sugar-sweetened beverages (SSB) and soft drinks. Sugar has high glycemic index (GI), meaning it enters the bloodstream easily. As a guide, these are the Glycemic Index Definitions:

- **High:** 70 and above
- **Moderate:** 56-69
- **Low:** 55 and below

Refined sugar has a GI of 65, which is near the high levels. This explains why, when drinking sugary beverages, people usually experience *sugar rush* followed by a *sugar crash*.

We cannot totally shun sugar, as carbohydrates is an essential macronutrient alongside protein and fats. Besides, nutrient-dense foods have natural sugars in them. The key is just to regulate the carbohydrates we eat and the added sugar that we consume, especially when they come in the form of empty calories.

As the *American Academy of Pediatrics* said: *"Sugars consumed in nutrient-poor foods and beverages are the primary problem to be addressed, not simply sugars themselves. Consumed within recommended calorie amounts, sweetness can offer an effective tool to promote consumption of nutrient-dense foods and beverages."*

Regulating Sugar

Moderation is the key. Below is a general guideline on how sugar fits into a healthy diet, based on *Dietary Guidelines for Americans 2010* and the *American Heart Association*.

✓ *45% to 60% carbohydrates/sugar/starch*
  ○ between 225 and 325 grams of carbohydrates a day
  ○ *added sugar* must only be 25 to 37.5 grams (9%)
    ▪ Men: 37.5 grams or 9 teaspoons (150 calories per day)

- Women: 25 grams or 6 teaspoons (100 calories per day)

Note: 1 tsp sugar = 4 grams = 15 calories
- ✓ **20% to 35% protein**
- ✓ **20% to 25% fat**

As gleaned from the ratios, it is wise to consume sugar with protein and fiber to slow down the entry of glucose in the bloodstream. As they say, eat your sugar, do not drink them. You can also use sugar-free sweeteners.

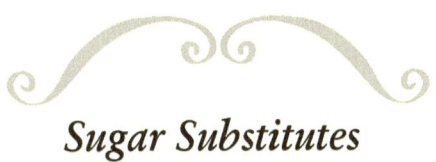

Sugar Substitutes

A sugar substitutes is any sweetener intended to replace regular sugar or sucrose. They are either natural or artificial. *Natural sweeteners* such as honey and coco sugar have more or less similar caloric content as regular sugar, while *artificial sweeteners* are often low-calorie. There are also other types: *modified sugar*, which are used often in processed food and which you should stay away from as much as possible due to their high glycemic index; and *sugar alcohols* which are good sugar substitutes.

Sugar substitutes, especially sugar alcohols and artificial sweeteners, are useful for diabetics and for people watching their sugar intake. But again, it must be in **moderation**. The rule of thumb is: You are okay if sugar substitutes such as artificial sweeteners satisfy your need for sweet taste or if they make you eat healthier by improving the taste of healthy food. But if those alternatives make you crave for more sugar, or if they make you consume more calories (for example by making you justify eating more), then look elsewhere or perhaps retrain your taste buds.

The next chapters will look at these various types of sugar substitutes.

MARY CONRAD

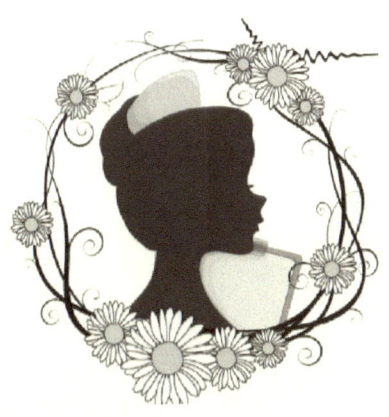

Chapter 2

Modified Sugar

This is the result when enzymes are used to convert starch to sugar, or when sugar is modified into syrups by heating or adding enzymes or chemicals. This type of sugar is widely used in processed and packaged foods. They have high glycemic index and, like regular sugar, may cause tooth decay among other health conditions. There are also other kinds such as agave syrup which were previously considered healthy alternatives, until recent studies showed negative side effects due to high fructose content.

The general rule for modified sugar is to use them in moderation, and include them in the count of the acceptable daily intake on added sugar.

Agave Syrup or Agave Nectar

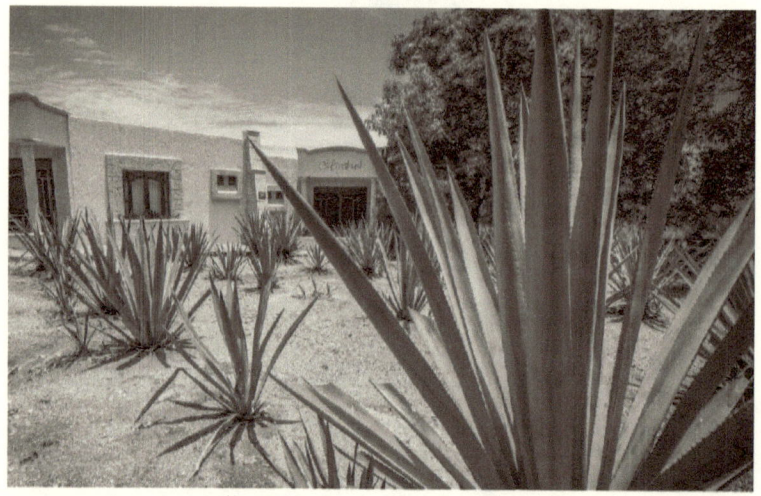

Source and Production: As the name suggests, it comes from agave, a cactus-looking succulent or water-storing plant from Mexico (it's the same plant from where tequila is made). The sap from the core of the plant is extracted, and enzyme-treated to become agave syrup. However, commercially-available agave syrup products are made using the starch of the giant root bulb, which is not that sweet, and which consists of about 50% inulin and 50% starch. This starch extract is hydrolyzed and treated with enzymes.

Profile: It is 50% sweeter than table sugar, hence only a small amount is needed. A teaspoon of agave syrup has 20 calories, but only half is required to achieve same level of sweetness as table sugar, cutting spoon-equivalent calories down to 10. By contrast, 1 tsp table sugar has 15 calories. Since agave nectar is in syrup form, it is also heavier than table sugar (7 grams per teaspoon, versus 4 grams of table sugar). Compared to honey, agave syrup is sweeter but less thick/viscous. It has notes of caramel.

Pros: It has fiber, prebiotics, and low glycemic index (15 vs 65 white sugar).

Cons: It is more expensive than regular sugar. There are also issues regarding its health/nutrition profile. *Weston A Price Foundation* dubs it as hydrolyzed inulin syrup. Though it has low GI, its fructose content is high (anywhere from 60% to 92%), hence it must be taken in moderation. Fructose is processed by the liver, so excessive intake can take a toll on the liver, and can lead to obesity. There are also other manufacturers that adulterate or extend agave syrup with high fructose corn syrup.

Usage*:* Use in moderation and in fewer amount. As a rule of thumb:
- ✓ In beverages: 1 tsp refined sugar = ½ tsp agave syrup
- ✓ When baking or cooking: 1 cup refined sugar = ⅔ cup agave syrup + reduce liquid by ¼ cup

Usual Brands: Volcanic Nectar Blue Agave, Nekutli, IIDEA, Agave in the Raw, Wholesome Sweeteners Organic Blue Agave Nectar, Madhava, Blue Green Agave Organic Nectar

Barley Malt Syrup

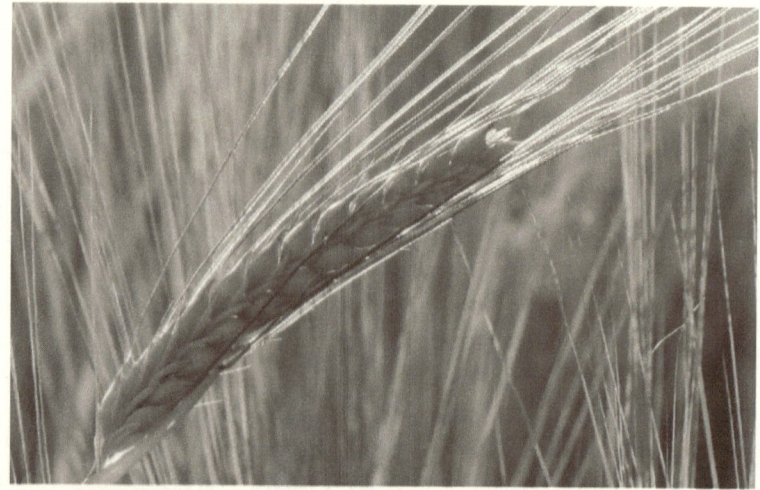

Source and Production: This is made by soaking and sprouting barley to make malt, then cooking it down to a thick, dark brown, sticky syrup. The enzyme that transforms the starch to sugar naturally occurs in the sprouted barley grains, making this a naturally modified type of sugar.

Profile: It has a rich, toasted taste and features the same texture as molasses, the byproduct of refined sugar. It is half as sweet as table sugar, hence requiring double the amount to achieve the same level of sweetness. Like agave syrup, it weighs more than table sugar (7 grams versus 4 grams of table sugar).

Pros: Made up of 60% maltose, its levels of sucrose and fructose are close to zero, making it low glycemic (42 versus 65 of table sugar). It is also rich in fiber, vitamins, and minerals. It is used to treat digestive problems such as constipation and irritable bowel movement.

Cons: It's more expensive than table sugar, and requires double dosage too. Calories per teaspoon is also similar with table sugar (16 to 22 calories per teaspoon versus 15 calories for table sugar), but again two servings are needed to achieve the same sweetness level. Also, since it is made from barley, it is not suitable for people with gluten intolerance.

Usage: Double the amount when using to replace white sugar. In its granulated form, it is a good substitute for brown sugar. Drizzle it on cereal, pancakes, popcorn, and roasted vegetables; or use in spice cakes, muffins, and whole grain breads. It is also used as an ingredient for brewing beer and wine.

Usual Brands: Eden, Barry Farm, Clearspring

Brown Rice Syrup

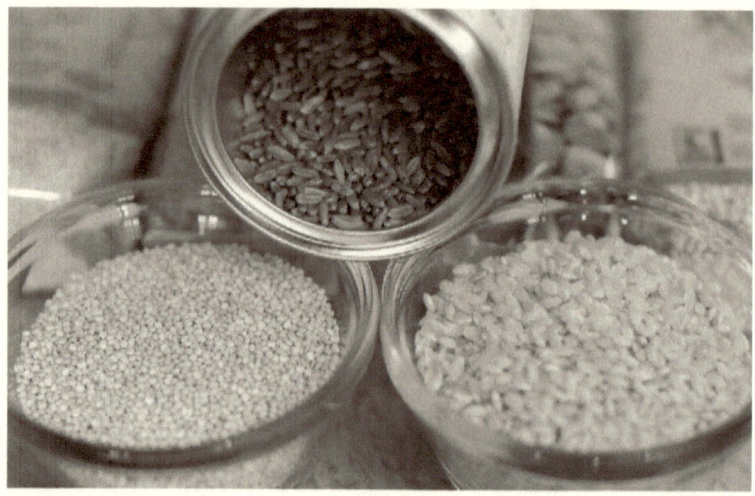

<u>**Source and Production**</u>: Brown whole grain rice is cooked with malt or sprouted barley, converting starch to sugar. The liquid is boiled until it becomes gooey and thick like honey.

<u>**Profile**</u>: It has a mild taste, similar with light honey, with notes of caramel and butterscotch. Like other sugar syrups, it is heavier than table sugar. Like Agave and Malt Syrups, each teaspoon weighs 7 grams. Its sweetness level and caloric profile is similar with those of Malt Syrup: half as sweet as table sugar with about the same level of calories per teaspoon.

<u>**Pros**</u>: Composed of 65% maltose and zero sucrose and fructose, it has low glycemic index (25). It is rich in vitamins and minerals including potassium, magnesium, and B vitamins.

<u>**Cons**</u>: As a complex carbohydrate, it is rather filling. However, its calorie content is high, requiring double the calories to achieve same level of sweetness as table sugar. It is also more expensive. Some products and brands use artificial enzymes, so it is wise to check the label when buying.

Usage: This is best to use in granola, muffins, brownies, breads, pancakes, and oatmeal. However, given its strong taste, it is not recommended for light desserts or baked items with light flavor as it can get overpowering.

Usual Brand: Lundberg, Rawseed, Ottogi

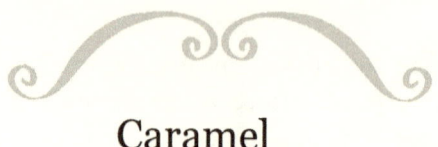

Caramel

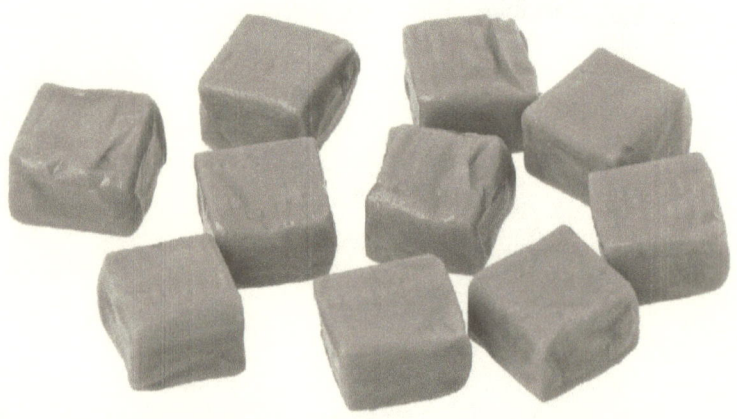

Source and Production: Caramel is made by heating sugar to 170°C. It can be made at home. Water and cream are added in other recipes. Caramel can be light or dark brown in color, depending on temperature and duration of heating.

Profile: Caramel has a distinct and pleasant taste. It adds color, flavor, and texture to food and beverages.

Pros: It tastes good.

Cons: It has the same sweetness index, glycemic level, and calories as table sugar. Like table sugar, it has no nutritive value.

Usage: Though seldom used as on its own, it is often used in cakes, ice cream, flans, and puddings. It is a common ingredient of fudge, toffee, cola, beer, and whiskey. It is also a popular add-on to coffee and chocolate.

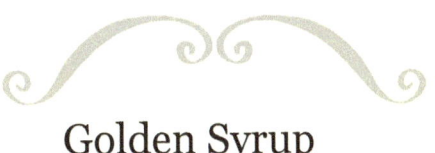

Golden Syrup

Source and Production: This comes from the same process that refines sugar. To make table sugar, sugarcane is boiled. Once sugar crystallizes, it is removed, then the process is repeated over again. One stage of this manufacturing produces the golden syrup. This byproduct was discovered by Abram Lyle in 1883.

Profile: Golden syrup contains 56% inverted sugar (27% fructose, 27% glucose, 2% other) and 44% sucrose. It is thick and has a rich and pleasant taste. It is also 10% sweeter than sugar.

Pros: Like other syrups, it is a rich and pleasant substitute to sugar in recipes.

Cons: It is just another form of refined sugar; hence it has similar caloric profile (15 grams per spoon-equivalent) and glycemic index (60) as table sugar. Unlike molasses, golden syrup is devoid of nutritional value.

Usage: Use it in baking tarts, puddings, and bars such as flapjacks, or in cooking savory sauces and dishes.

Other Common Names: Partially Inverted Refiners Syrup

Usual Brands: Tate & Lyle's Golden Syrup (titleholder as Guinness world's oldest branding/packaging)

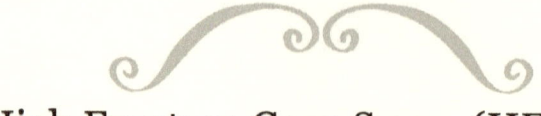

High Fructose Corn Syrup (HFCS)

Source and Production: This is made by treating cornstarch with enzyme. It is not commercially-available, but it is widely used in packaged consumer goods.

Profile: It is 20% sweeter than sugar. Aside from this, they taste the same. It was invented in the 1950s, produced for industrial use in the 1970s, and since then has become a hit among manufacturers because it is 50% cheaper than table sugar. It is widely used in USA and all over the world, except in the European Union. Consumers have started to veer away from this, in the similar way that they vilified hydrogenated fats and trans-fat in the past years.

Pros: Useful for manufacturers because it is more economical, while retaining the desired properties of table sugar (i.e. sweet taste, browns when heated, good color, feeds yeast, thickens, stabilizes, and prolongs shelf life of processed food).

Cons: It has similar caloric profile (13 per spoon-equivalent) and glycemic index (58) as table sugar. Unlike table sugar which is 50-50 fructose and glucose, HFCS contains 55% fructose, 42% glucose, and 3% other sugar. This seemingly small imbalance can wreak havoc on metabolism, especially when compounded by overconsumption. Several studies have provided some interesting data on HFCS:

- A study conducted in Princeton University found that intake of this sugar can cause fat accumulation by 300% compared to fruit derived sugar. This result indicates a higher chance of developing obesity. A similar study supports this and adds that excessive consumption (such as those found in beverages) can elevate triglyceride levels (bad cholesterol), which in turn would eventually develop into plaques on the arterial walls (atherosclerosis).

- It also increases the risk of developing Type-2 Diabetes.
- There are studies which indicate that HCFS is metabolized in the liver. Consistent consumption over a period of time could increase the development of fatty liver
- Although it may seem a little controversial, there's a certain study which found that there were high levels of mercury in over 50% of random samples taken.

Usage: It might be good to avoid this modified sugar. When buying food in supermarkets, read the label to check for the presence and level of HFCS.

Other Common Names: Isoglucose, Glucose Fructose Syrup, Corn Sugar

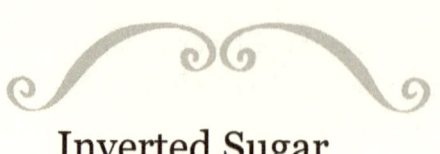

Inverted Sugar

Source and Production: This is made by boiling table sugar (1kg) and water (½L) with a bit of acid such as citric acid or cream of tartar (1g). Baking soda (½g) can also be added to neutralize the acidity.

Profile: It is 20% sweeter than table sugar. In a way, it is like HFCS but made with table sugar, which is from sugarcane or sugar beets. It also has a lower fructose level versus HFCS. Inverted sugar contains 37.5% fructose (vs 55% in HFCS), 37.5% glucose, 2.5% sucrose, 22.4% water, and 0.1% ash.

Pros: Good taste and texture. It is also hygroscopic or moisture-absorbing, prolonging shelf life while maintaining moistness and consistency. Inverted sugar can add flavor and texture to food – very useful for cooking and for professional chefs. It's used extensively in the food industry to control texture and improve shelf life of manufactured food products.

Cons: It has similar caloric profile (14 per spoon-equivalent) and glycemic index (60) as table sugar. It is just another form of sugar, and is like high fructose corn syrup albeit made from cane or beet. Avoiding excessive consumption is important. Also, keep in mind that inverted sugar isn't suited for diabetics.

Usage: It is used in soft centers of chocolates, candies, marzipan, and liquors. Popular example is Cadbury Creme Egg. It is also used by professional chefs.

Other Common Names: Invert Sugar, Invert Syrup

Summary

Modified Sugar	Pros	Cons	Potential Side Effects of Use
Agave Syrup or Agave Nectar	Contains prebiotics	High levels of fructose	Not advised for those with liver problems and diabetes.
Barley Malt Syrup	Levels of sucrose and fructose are close to zero, making it low glycemic and rich in fiber, vitamins, and minerals	Expensive and requires more servings to achieve the sweetness of table sugar	Not advised for those with gluten intolerance.
Brown Rice Syrup	Low glycemic index (25). It is rich in vitamins and minerals including potassium, magnesium, and B vitamins.	Calorie content is high, requiring double the calories to achieve same level of sweetness as table sugar.	Careful calorie count for those with diabetes.
Caramel	Tastes good.	No nutritive value	Not advised for diabetics
Golden Syrup	It's a different form of refined sugar.	It has the same disadvantages as refined sugar.	Not advised for diabetics
High	Similar to	Can cause	Long-term

Fructose Corn Syrup (HFCS)	table sugar in terms of taste, texture and properties	potential metabolic problems. Not for diabetics	use can lead to cardiac problems and obesity.
Inverted Sugar	Good taste and texture. Can prolong shelf life when added to food.	Calorie index is the same as table sugar.	Not advised for diabetics.

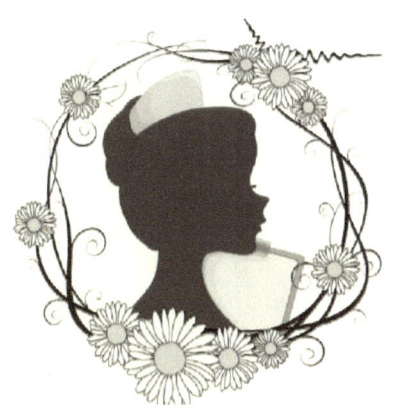

Chapter 3

Natural Sugar Substitutes

Natural sugar substitutes are sweeteners that come from alternative plant sources. They can be caloric or zero calorie.

The great thing about this sweetener is they are usually more nutritious than regular sugar. Honey is a great example of a natural sweetener that has several uses with both antibacterial properties and nutritional value. There are forms of these sugars that doesn't undergo any processing, which saves the worry of additives. However, there are a few under this classification that is being manufactured and processed, so reading the labels is a must. This is very common for powder forms of natural sweeteners such as stevia.

Caloric Natural Sugar Substitutes

These sugar extracts contain more or less the same amount of calories as refined sugar. However, they have more fiber, soluble and insoluble alike, helping regulate blood sugar. Generally, they also have lower glycemic index, and hence are not as addictive as refined sugar.

Aside from this, they contain other nutrients such as potassium, sodium, magnesium, and B vitamins. Unlike refined sugar, they tend to have fewer chemical residues from manufacturing and refining because they are naturally-extracted from plant sources.

Many of these sweeteners have been around and used by indigenous people even before the discovery of refined sugar, and some have been used for their medicinal properties.

Like regular sugar though, when taken in excessive amounts, they are harmful to the teeth, among other medical conditions. As a general rule, caloric natural sweeteners must be taken into account when it comes to the acceptable daily intake of added sugar.

The following are the different kinds of caloric natural sweeteners in alphabetical order:

Cane Juice

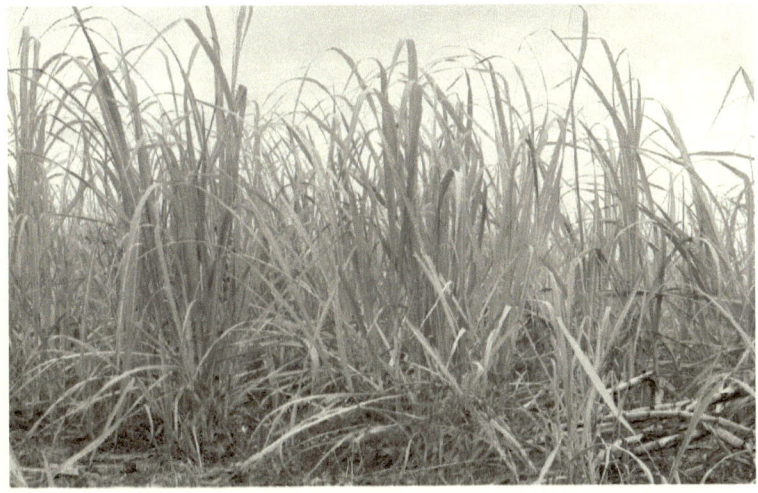

Source and Production: This is made by crushing sugarcane. In essence, sucrose and water are just separated from the fiber/pulp.

Profile: It is as sweet as table sugar. In a way, it is just a fruit juice form of table sugar.

Pros: It has lower glycemic index (43) than table sugar, while having the same level of sweetness. It doesn't have any nutritional value but in small amounts it is a bit healthier than table sugar. The less it is processed the better it is.

Cons: Roughly the same number of calories (16) as table sugar.

Usage: It is usually sold as a drink in itself to quench thirst. It is too watery to be used as a sweetener.

Other Common Names: Evaporated Cane Juice, Cane Juice Concentrate

Coconut Palm Sugar

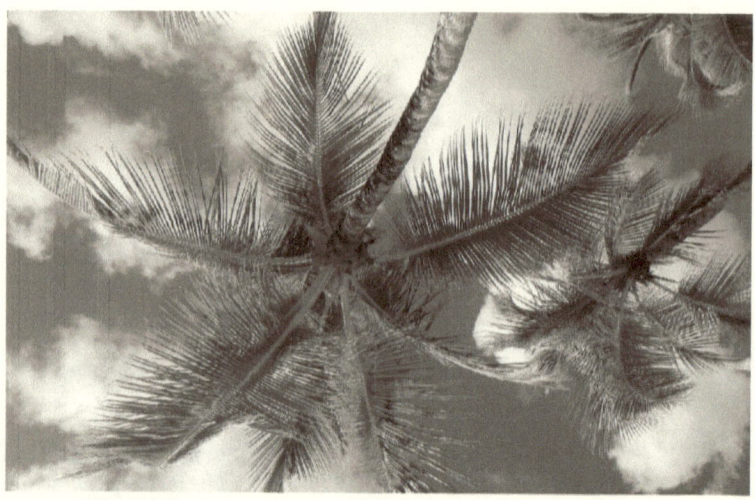

Source and Production: It comes from the sap of the flower buds of the coconut palm tree. This liquid nectar is collected and boiled, resulting to water evaporation and yielding granulated sugar. No chemicals or enzymes are added.

Profile*:* Technically, it has the same level of sweetness as sugar, but its unique roasted and nutty taste makes some consumers feel that it is less sweet.

Pros*:* It has lower glycemic index (35 to 50) versus table sugar, and contains more vitamins and minerals such as iron, zinc, calcium, magnesium, potassium, and B vitamins. Since it is not refined with enzymes, it is a truly natural alternative, unlike agave and other syrups. It is also considered sustainably-grown, harvested, and manufactured.

Cons*:* It is more expensive than table sugar. It also has no fiber, and it is still sugar, and hence must be taken in moderation.

Usage*:* Use in beverages, especially coffee. The taste might not suit teas. It is also good to use in baking and cooking. It goes well with curries and savory dishes and sauces, and adds depth and richness to baked goods such as brownies.

Other Common Names: Coco Sugar, Coconut Sugar

Usual Brands*:* Sweet Tree, Palm Nectar Organics, Wholesome Sweeteners, Tropical Sweet, Madhava Sweeteners, Coco Natura, Bob's Red Mill, Cocovie Naturals

Date Sugar

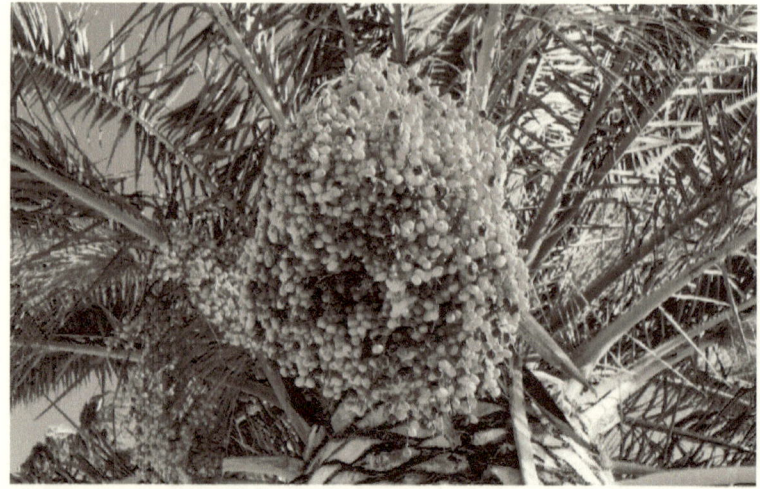

<u>Source and Production</u>: This comes from dates, fruits of date palm trees. It is made by dehydrating dates and grinding them. This can be made at home. To dry the dates, use a dehydrator, bake in an oven, or dry out in the sun. To grind, use a food processor or a coffee/nut grinder.

<u>Profile</u>: This is slightly sweeter than white sugar, so less is required. It has a slightly thicker consistency than sugar.

<u>Pros</u>: This has a low glycemic index (46 to 55). It is also rich in fiber and vitamins. Like coconut sugar, date sugar is also all-natural as chemicals are not required to process it. Nonetheless, check the label when buying date sugar in groceries.

<u>Cons</u>: Unlike coco sugar, date sugar does not dissolve, so do not stir it in beverages, even hot ones, as the drink will be grainy. It is also not recommended for light desserts or baked items with light flavor as date sugar can get overpowering. It is also more expensive than regular sugar.

Usage: Use it in dishes where you would appreciate its richness such as topping for oats, rub or marinade for meat, sugar half-replacement in brownies and cookies, and sweetener for sauces. Since it is sweeter than sugar, you'll have to make the necessary adjustments: 1 cup refined sugar = ⅔ cup date sugar.

Usual Brands: Bob's Red Mill, Chatfield's, Now Foods, Date Lady

Other Variations: Date sugar is also available in the form of syrup puréed/mashed with honey called *silan* or date honey, popular in Mediterranean cuisine.

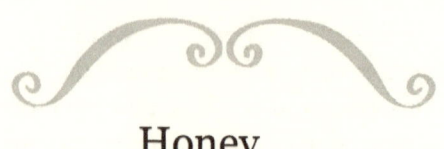

Honey

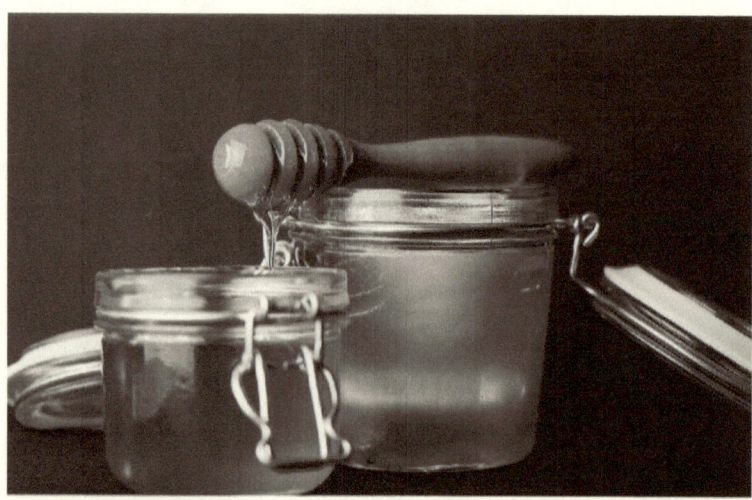

Source and Production: Dubbed as the oldest sweetener, honey is produced by worker bees that collect nectar from flowers. They have natural enzymes that transform nectar to honey. Each bee produces about $^1/_{10}$ teaspoon honey in its 6-week lifespan.

Profile: Honey is made of 41% fructose, 36% glucose, 18% water, 3% galactose, 1.8% maltose, and 0.2% ash. It is 10% sweeter than granulated sugar. While honey comes mostly in syrup, it is also available in solid form.

Pros: It is rich in iron, zinc, calcium, potassium, vitamin B6, riboflavin, niacin, and antioxidants. It also promotes growth of healthy bacteria in the digestive system. Honey is known for its medicinal, anti-bacterial, and antiseptic qualities. People use it to soothe sore throat and heal infection.

Cons: It is more expensive than regular sugar. It is also high glycemic (50-55) and must be consumed in moderation.

Usage: There are many variations of honey. Choose raw honey from trusted sources. Raw honey, 100% honey, or unfiltered honey may contain solids called bee pollen.

Specific Variants: Ulmo Honey (Chile), Manuka Honey (New Zealand)

Usual Brands: Nature Nate's, Y.S. Eco Bee Farms, Honest, Kirkland, Honey Tree's

Lucuma Powder

Source and Production: This comes from the lucuma fruit (native to Peru), also known as eggfruit or Incan gold due to its yolk-like color. It is made by dehydrating and grinding the fruit.

Profile: The fruit tastes like maple syrup with notes of yam or sweet potato, while the dried powder is reminiscent of goji berries and apricots. It adds a caramel taste and rich texture to food and beverages.

Pros: As a complex carbohydrate, it is rich in iron, zinc, potassium, calcium, magnesium, vitamin B3, beta carotene, and fiber. It also has low glycemic index (25).

Cons: It is more expensive than refined sugar. Like date sugar, it also does not dissolve completely in liquid, resulting to grainy beverages.

Usage: It is very versatile and can be used in cooking, baking, as well as in preparing smoothies and blended drinks.

Usual Brands: Navitas Naturals, Sunfood, Nua Naturals

Maple Syrup

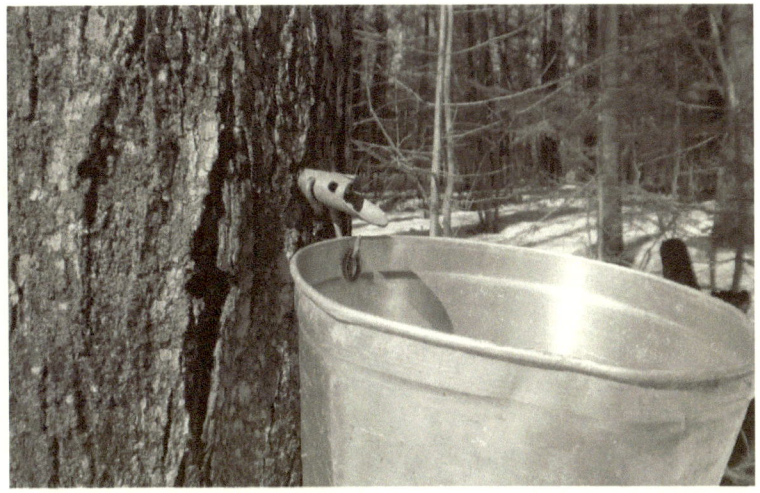

Source and Production: Widely-produced especially in Canada, maple syrup is extracted from maple trees. To get the sap, a small hole is drilled into the tree to allow the sap to flow out. The sap is boiled into a concentrated, sticky syrup.

Profile: It is as sweet as table sugar, and thinner than honey.

Pros: Since no chemicals or enzymes are added, it is a pure and natural product. It is rich in antioxidants, zinc, manganese, and B vitamins. It also has a slightly lower glycemic index (54) than sugar.

Cons: Pure maple syrup is expensive. It also has different grades. Be wary of cheap versions, especially those served in restaurants that usually have high fructose corn syrup and food coloring. Given its moderate GI, it is not suitable for diabetics.

Usage: Aside from using it as pancake drizzle, try adding it to meat glazes and rubs, sauces, and desserts such as ice cream. It is also available in granulated form.

Usual Brands: Canadian Finest, Slopeside Syrup, Fadden's, Crown, Hilltop Boilers, Brown Family Farm, Camp, Kirkland, Trader Joe's, Mrs. Butterworth's, Log Cabin

Molasses

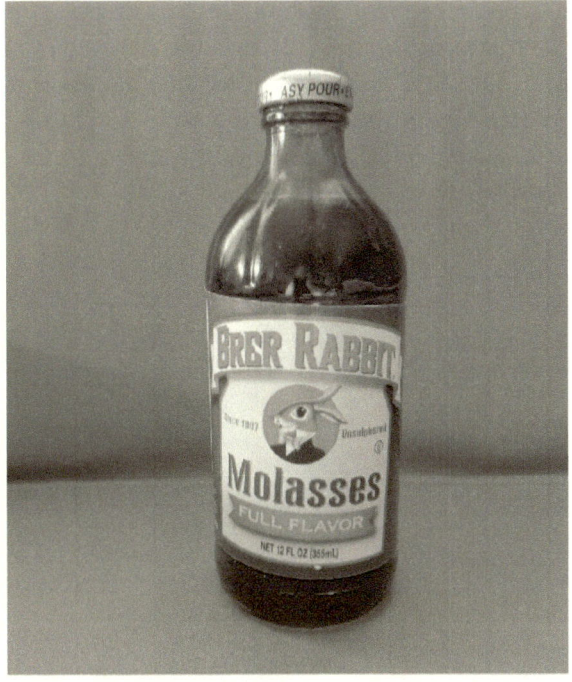

Source and Production: This is the byproduct when sugarcane is processed to refined sugar – the leftover goodness, as some say. Sugarcane's deep roots absorb nutrients from soil, hence cane molasses has good flavor and plenty of nutrients. This cannot be said for beet molasses which is used as cattle feed and not suitable for human consumption due to poor taste.

Profile: Molasses is a thick dark syrup that's 20% less sweet than sugar, and has a strong flavor akin to licorice.

Pros*:* It is rich in magnesium, iron, potassium, calcium, copper, zinc, and B vitamins. As an iron-rich food, it is recommended for people with anemia. It also has medicinal uses, providing relief from premenstrual syndrome and helping in the management of other conditions such as obesity and acne.

Cons: Due to its high glycemic index (60), it is not suitable for diabetics.

Usage: It is good for baking and in making savory sauces. Because of its strong flavor, it is not meant for recipes calling for light flavor. Molasses is also used in making alcoholic drinks such as rum. Like maple syrup, molasses also comes in grades. Some grades have added sulfur dioxide, while others contain up to 20% fructose. Check the label when buying molasses.

Other Common Names: Blackstrap Molasses, Black Treacle

Usual Brands: Golden Barrel, Plantation, Wholesome Sweeteners, Grandma's, Aunt Patty's, Meridian

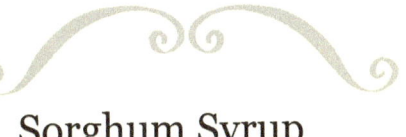

Sorghum Syrup

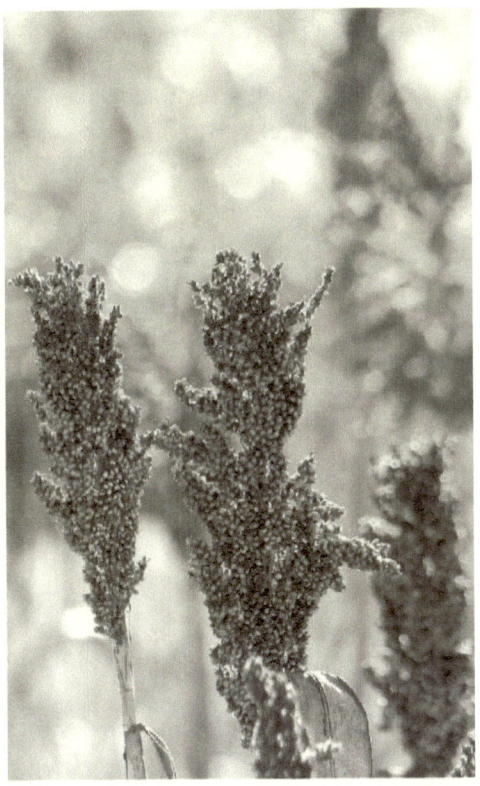

Source and Production: This is made from sweet sorghum cane, a grass native to Africa. The stems are crushed, and the juice extracted, filtered, and boiled until it becomes a thick syrup. No chemicals or enzymes are needed.

Profile: The dark brown syrup is 10% sweeter than refined sugar, and as thick as honey. It also has a pleasantly sour taste like molasses. Its typical composition is 46% sucrose, 22.5% water, 16% glucose, 13% fructose, and 2.5% ash.

Pros: It is rich in calcium, magnesium, manganese, potassium, zinc, and B vitamins, with low glycemic index (50).

Cons: Since it is mostly sucrose, it must be taken in moderation. Moreover, it is quite expensive and getting scarce. Diabetics can consume this as long as they count it against their allowable added sugar.

Usage: It is traditionally used as a drizzle over hot biscuits. Use it the same way as honey and other syrups.

Other Common Names: Kentucky's Maple Syrup, Sorghum Molasses

Usual Brands: Golden Barrel, Muddy Pond, Bourbon Barrel Foods

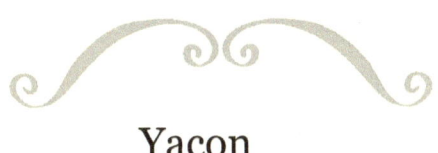

Yacon

Source and Production: This is made from Yacon tuber, also known as Peruvian ground apple native to South America, which tastes like apple but sweeter. It is made the same way as Sorghum Syrup but using the roots of the tuber. The Yacon roots are ground to extract juice then heat-treated until a syrup is formed.

Profile: The syrup tastes like caramel and fig, and half as sweet as sugar.

Pros: Its sweetness comes from carbohydrate Fructo-Oligosaccharides (FOS), an insoluble fiber. It has high concentration of inulin, a complex sugar, hence it takes long to break down, regulating blood sugar. It also regulates insulin and cholesterol levels. It is rich in potassium, calcium, phosphorous, iron, and amino acids. As a prebiotic, it promotes the growth of beneficial gut bacteria and can relieve constipation. It has almost zero GI (1), and only has half to a third of the calories of regular sugar. Packed with nutrients and health benefits, it is considered a superfood.

Cons: Initial and excessive intake can cause bloating. It is also expensive.

Usage: It is not used as a sweetener per se, but more for its health benefits.

Other Common Names: Yacon Syrup, Yacon Nectar

Usual Brands: Peruvian Naturals, Nature Botanical Farms

Zero-Calorie Natural Sugar Substitutes

Before, the only zero-calorie sweeteners available in the mainstream market are artificial ones. But recent years saw the popularization of naturally zero-calorie alternatives from Africa, South America, and Asia.

These zero-calorie sugar substitutes also have zero glycemic index, making them suitable for diabetics. Moreover, they do not cause tooth decay. The downside is that they tend to taste quite differently from refined sugar, or have an aftertaste that may need some getting used to. Aside from the struggle of acquired taste, they also lean more on the expensive side.

Most of these zero-calorie natural sweeteners do not have upper limits yet on how much to consume, but as a general rule, use them in moderation as you would do with regular sugar. Do not overconsume just because it is zero-calorie.

Below are four common zero-calorie sweeteners, although there are other types which are not yet FDA-approved or not yet commercially-available worldwide, such as *Brazzein* and *Pentadin* (Oubli Climbing Plant, West Africa), *Curculin* (Curculigo Latifolia fruit, Malaysia), *Monellin* (Serendipity Berry, Central and West Africa), and *Thaumatin* (Katemfe Fruit, Sudan; EU-approved as E957).

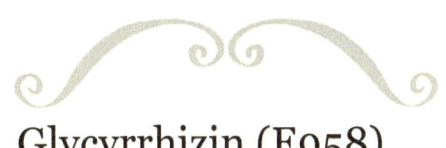

Glycyrrhizin (E958)

Source and Production: This is extracted from the roots of licorice. Glycyrrhizin is used mostly by food and pharmaceutical companies to flavor candies and medicine.

Profile: It has a strong licorice flavor and aftertaste, and is 50 times sweeter than sugar.

Pros: It has medicinal qualities to treat ulcers and is also good as an expectorant for coughs.

Cons: Excessive intake may worsen hypertension. Limit consumption to 100mg per day.

Usage: Not used by regular consumers as sweetener, but manufacturers use it in candies, chewing gum, lozenges, and medicine to achieve a licorice flavor. It is also used as a toothpaste ingredient, as well as to sweeten tea, tobacco, and processed food.

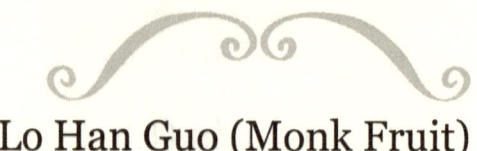

Lo Han Guo (Monk Fruit)

Source and Production: This is extracted from Lo Han Guo, a plant native to Guangxi, China. The monk fruit is crushed and infused with hot water, then heat-treated to extract the sweetness that comes from mogroside in the meat of the fruit.

Profile: The resulting light-brown powder is 300 times sweeter than sugar, so less is required. It also tastes better than Stevia, though some would say it has an off aftertaste. It is usually mixed with other types of sugar to balance the sweetness and taste.

Pros: It has zero calorie and zero glycemic index. The Chinese have used it in the past 800 years as a medicine for sore throat, cough, and fever. It also serves as an antioxidant, and lowers blood sugar levels.

Cons: None, but there's a need for more studies as it is a relatively new entrant to the sugar substitute market, despite it being used for many years in China.

Usual Brands: BioVittoria (New Zealand), Tate and Lyle (UK), Neway Natural's Sweet Sensation (with maltitol), Splenda's Nectresse (with Erythritol), Monk Fruit in the Raw (with dextrose), Lakanto (with Erythritol)

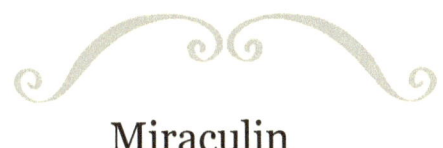

Miraculin

Source and Production: This is harvested from the fleshy meat of Miracle Fruit, a berry used in West Africa for hundreds of years.

Profile: It is actually not sweet at all, but it alters the taste buds for a period of time (15-60 mins), making sour foods taste sweet. It is available as freeze-dried berries, tablets, or granules.

Pros: It has zero calories and zero glycemic index. This is very suitable for diabetics. It is also used in medicine to improve palatability. It has also been used to relieve the side effect of Chemotherapy medication that makes food taste metallic.

Cons: Miraculin just alters the perception of taste, not actual taste and chemistry. Take miraculin in moderation to avoid stomach irritation, and to still enjoy the natural flavor of food. Effects can last up to 18 hours.

Usual Sources: BioResources International, Inc. (BRI), Miracle Fruit Express (Sen Yuh Farm Science Company, Taiwan), Miracle Fruit Farm (Miami)

Stevia

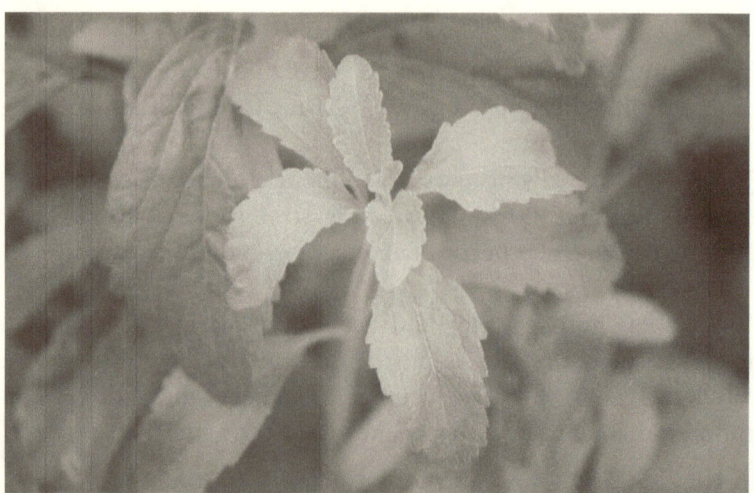

Source and Production: This is the first natural zero calorie sugar to enter the mainstream market. It comes from the Stevia rebaudiana plant/herb from South America, specifically Paraguay, where it has been used for centuries. The Japanese has been using it since the 1970s.

Profile*:* The fine powder is 300 times sweeter than sugar, and much less needs to be used. It is also available in other forms such as liquid concentrated extract called Stevioside (EU-approved as E960), tabletop packets, liquid drops, dissolvable tablets, and spoonable products.

Pros*:* It has zero calories and zero carbohydrates, thus it does not raise blood sugar. It also alleviates high blood pressure, and has anti-inflammatory properties.

Cons*:* It has a slight aftertaste described as bitter, licorice-like, and metallic. There have been instances where stevia manufacturers have exploited this sweetener during processing by adding additives. In some instances, maltodextrin, which is derived from cornstarch is added to form the clear white powder. Check the labels and research on the brand before purchase.

Usage: Use it to replace sugar in drinks and dishes. Manufacturers also use it in diet sodas and sports drinks.

Usual Brands: NuNaturals, SweetLeaf, Truvia, Pure Via, Now Foods, Stevia in the Raw

Summary

Caloric Natural Sugar Substitute	Pros	Cons	Possible Side Effects
Cane Juice	It's slightly healthier that table sugar in small amounts	It has the same caloric value as table sugar	Long term use in high amounts can cause liver problems.
Coconut Palm Sugar	Same sweetness of sugar with a nutty flavor and has nutritive value	It still needs to be taken in moderation.	It can still raise blood sugar levels
Date Sugar	Lower glycemic index compared to table sugar and has more nutritive value	It doesn't dissolve very well	It can still raise blood sugar levels
Honey	Has medicinal properties and more natural	Must be consumed in moderation	It can still raise blood sugar levels
Lucuma Powder	More nutritive value compared to table sugar	Doesn't dissolve completely in water	Can help with deficiencies but requires moderation.
Maple Syrup	It's healthier compared to	Expensive and comes in	It requires moderation

	tale sugar with a slightly lower glycemic index	different grades.	especially for those with diabetes
Molasses	Rich in iron and can relieve PMS	Not for diabetics	Can help with iron deficiency but needs moderation since it can elevate blood glucose levels.
Sorghum Syrup	Rich in nutrients	Expensive and getting scarce.	Can be consumed by diabetics in their daily allowable sugar intake
Yacon	It is a prebiotic which promotes gut health	Excessive intake causes bloating	Not to be consumed excessively since it can cause an increase in blood sugar levels. It is also broken down by the liver.

Zero-Calorie NSS	Pros	Cons	Possible Effects of Use
Glycyrrhizin (E958)	Used to treat ulcers and as an expectorant	Can worsen hypertension	It should be used with caution by those with hypertension and heart problems.
Lo Han Guo	Has medicinal uses	None so far	Further studies are needed
Miraculin	Helps alleviate chemotherapy side effects in food taste	It only alters taste perception and	Too much consumption of different food such as spicy or sour since they taste sweet.
Stevia	It is sweeter than sugar without calories and carbohydrates	Has a bitter aftertaste	Can cause nausea

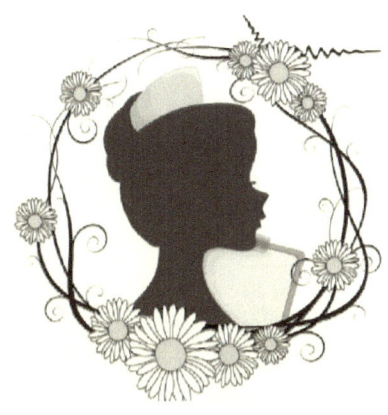

Chapter 4

Artificial Sugar Substitutes

Artificial sweeteners are made from chemicals. Most of them were discovered by accident in laboratories. When a packaged food or beverage says that it is sugar-free or diet, it most likely contains these artificial sweeteners.

While these artificial sweeteners have zero calories and are harmless to the teeth, they are also non-nutritive – and recent studies suggest that they have a negative effect on gut flora, and may lead to a slew of metabolic problems. For now, while further studies are yet to provide conclusive results, what we know is that some are safe while others need to be regulated, as excessive and prolonged use may be harmful to the body.

Sugar enthusiast Arthur McCooey lists Saccharin and Cyclamate as the safest kinds, and Sucralose and Aspartame as the least safe. Many other medical sources and consumer-oriented groups share similar sentiments.

These artificial sugar substitutes are considered high-intensity sweeteners as they are 40 to 20,000 times sweeter than ordinary sugar. Given the high levels of sweetness, only tiny amounts are needed – so miniscule that acceptable daily intake (ADI) levels are in milligrams, with cans of sodas as easy reference for recommended amount. You may be surprised that the acceptable daily intake for artificial sweeteners can translate to 36 to 800 cans of diet soda. But do you really need/want to consume this much?

The general recommendation is to use safe artificial sweeteners if there is a medical condition, such as diabetes or celiac disease, that prohibits the individual from taking regular sugar and its natural substitutes. These artificial sweeteners can also aid in weight management provided that they are consumed in moderation and taken as a part of a healthy lifestyle.

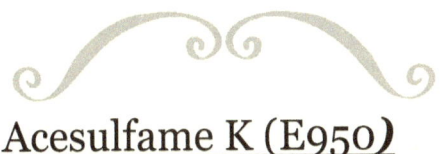

Acesulfame K (E950)

Source and Production: This is made by combining acetoacetic acid with potassium. The result is a stable and sweet crystalline substance. This was discovered by accident in 1967 by chemist Karl Clauss. He dipped his fingers into some chemicals in the laboratory. Later, he had to pick a piece of paper, and he licked his fingers to do so. He was surprised with the very sweet taste.

Profile: This is 200 times sweeter than sugar with a bit of bitter aftertaste, which is balanced when mixed with other sweeteners, resulting to combinations such as Aspartame-Acesulfame Salt.

Pros: It has zero glycemic index and zero calories. It is also cheap and heat-stable; hence it is used in many processed foods. The body does not metabolize or absorb this sweetener. It just passes through the gut and excreted in its unchanged state.

Cons: Consumer group *Center for Science in the Public Interest* (CSPI) has raised the red flag on Acesulfame K's carcinogenic or cancer-causing component, methylene chloride. Further studies have yet to provide conclusive evidence. There have been studies that state that this sweetener may interrupt the normal metabolic process as well as raise blood sugar levels. Some have also questioned the effect of this sugar to early fetal development.

This sugar is often mixed with aspartame and sucralose to mask the bitter aftertaste.

Usage: It has been USFDA-approved since 1988, GRAS in 2003, and in EU as E950. FDA set the acceptable daily intake (ADI) at 15mg/kg (mg per kg of body weight). This means, a 70kg person must not consume more than 1,050mg or 1.05g of Acesulfame K. For reference, Coke Zero has 31mg Acesulfame K and 58mg

Aspartame. This does not mean that you should load up on Coke Zero and Acesulfame K though.

<u>Other Common Names:</u> Ace K, Acesulfame Potassium

<u>Usual Brands</u>: Sunett, Sweet One

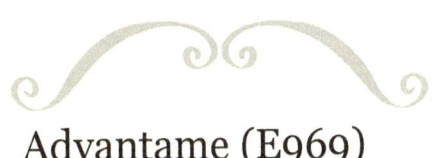

Advantame (E969)

Source and Production: This newest artificial sweetener made by Ajinomoto Japan in 2014 is produced by synthesizing aspartame and isovanillin.

Profile: It is 20,000 times sweeter than regular sugar. Very small amounts are needed, making it a very cheap alternative to sugar and HFCN. It is not just a sweetener, but a flavor enhancer too.

Pros: It has zero glycemic index and zero calories. Though it contains aspartame which is harmful to the body, only a small amount is needed, hence the negative effect is negligible.

Cons: It is not yet branded and not yet available to consumers. There are claims that just like aspartame, the potential adverse effects of this sweetener outweigh the benefits. Some believe that further studies should be made to ensure the safety of this for consumers.

Usage: It was USFDA-approved last 2014, in EU as 969, and also in Australia and New Zealand. Ironically, it is not yet approved in Japan. It is also endorsed by consumer group CSPI, along with Neotame. Acceptable daily intake is 32.8mg/kg. For a 70kg person, this would translate to a maximum of 2,296mg or 2.3g or 800 cans of advantame-sweetened soda.

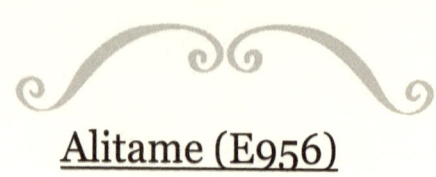

Alitame (E956)

Source and Production: This was developed by Pfizer in the early 1980s. It contains aspartic acid (present in Aspartame also) and alanine. In 2008, Danisco stopped production due to increased costs of raw materials.

Profile: It is 2,000 times sweeter than sugar, with no aftertaste. It's more heat stable versus its predecessor, Aspartame.

Pros: It is zero calorie and zero GI, and suitable for diabetics as well as those with phenylketonuria (PKU).

Cons: Given the cease in production, it is difficult to obtain in the market.

Usage: Approved in Mexico, China, Australia, and in EU as E956. Not yet approved by US FDA.

Usual Brand: Aclame

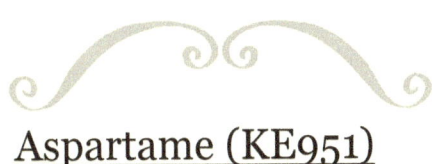

Aspartame (KE951)

Source and Production: It was discovered in 1965 by Searle chemist James M. Schlatter while he was assessing an anti-ulcer drug. Like how Clauss discovered Acesulfame K, Schlatter licked his finger to pick up a piece of paper and ended up tasting something sweet. Aspartame contains 40% Aspartic Acid, 50% Phenylalanine, and 10% Methanol. The patent expired in 1992, so aspartame is now widely and cheaply manufactured in China. It is usually combined with acesulfame-K to balance out the aftertaste.

Profile: This is 200 times as sweet as sugar. As a protein, each gram of it has 4 calories, but since it is very sweet, the serving amount has almost zero calories.

Pros: It has zero calories per serving and zero GI. It is also very cheap to produce and comes in various brands.

Cons: It has aftertaste described as cloying, bitter, and off. It isn't recommended for cooking because it breaks down in heat, reducing sweetness. Given its sensitivity to heat, it has poor shelf life especially in tropical and warm weather. It is also a controversial product due to customer complaints on side effects such as dizziness, headache, and blurred vision. People with phenylketonuria (PKU) cannot metabolize one of its components, phenylalanine. In fact, phenylalanine and methanol are toxic in high doses.

Usage: This is used in diet soft drinks and other low-calorie food, although manufacturers are exploring other alternatives due to customer concerns. It has been FDA-approved since 1996 but products must have a warning on phenylalanine content. EU approved it in 1994 as E951. Acceptable daily intake is 50mg/kg or 37 cans of aspartame-sweetened soda. But given the safety issues, it might be wise to use other sweeteners instead.

Other Common Names: *APM, Aspartyl Phenylalanine Methyl Ester, Blue Packets*

Usual Brands: NutraSweet, Equal, Canderel, AminoSweet, NatraTaste, Spoonful, Equal-Measure, Sugar Twin, Blue, Benevia

Aspartame-Acesulfame Salt (E962)

Source and Production: This was invented by Dr. John Fry in 1995. It is made by combining 64% Aspartame and 36% Acesulfame K in an acidic solution to crystallize, removing water and potassium in the process, and resulting to a fine powder or dry salt. In essence, Aspartame replaces the potassium component of Acesulfame K.

Profile: It is 350 times sweeter than sugar. It has 3 calories per gram, but since only a minimal amount is needed, it has almost zero calories per serving.

Pros: It has zero calories and zero GI. It also has good storage life, is heat stable, and does not absorb moisture.

Cons: While it is good for diabetics, its aspartame component makes it unsuitable for those with PKU. There are also reports on its side effects similar to those from aspartame consumption such as headache and nausea.

Usage: It is approved for use in USA and EU. Acceptable daily intake is 50mg/kg or 36 cans of soda sweetened with it. It's used in soft drinks and other food items. However, given customer complaints on aspartame content, manufacturers are exploring other alternatives. It may be a good choice to follow suit.

Usual Brand: Twinsweet

Cyclamate (E952, Sodium Cyclamate)

Source and Production: This is the second oldest artificial sugar substitute, the oldest being saccharin. The second oldest used to be Dulcin discovered in 1884, but it is not sold anymore. Cyclamate was discovered by accident in 1937 by a University of Illinois graduate student Michael Sveda. He was working on a fever medication when he brushed his lips with his unwashed hand and tasted something sweet.

Profile: This is the least potent of artificial sweeteners, as it is only 40 times sweeter than sugar. It has no aftertaste, and hence is usually mixed with saccharin (10 parts Cyclamate with 1 part Saccharin).

Pros: With zero calories and GI, it is okay for diabetics. It is also cheap.

Cons: It got a bad reputation in the late 1960s, when experiment rodents developed bladder tumors after having been fed large quantities of cyclamate for an extended period (equivalent of 350 cans of diet soda per day). Aside from this though, there were no human reports of side effects, unlike with Aspartame.

Usage: It was approved by US FDA in 1958, but this was revoked and the product banned in 1969 up to today. Given its status, ADI guidelines are not set, but it is recommended to take the product in moderation like other sugar types. It is approved in 50 other countries, including EU as E952.

Usual Brand: Sucaryl

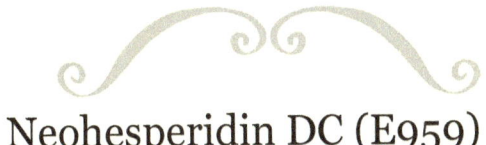

Neohesperidin DC (E959)

Source and Production: This was developed in the 1960s by the US Department of Agriculture as part of the endeavor to minimize the bitterness of citrus juices. Neohesperidin, derived from bitter oranges, is treated with potassium hydroxide or other strong base substances then hydrogenated.

Profile*:* It is 1,000 times sweeter than sugar with a sweet aftertaste that can be cloying. It is used more as a flavor enhancer instead of sweetener. Specifically, it masks bitter flavors and brings out subtle flavors of food and drinks.

Pros*:* It has zero GI and calories, hence making it suitable for diabetics. It is also heat-stable and pH-stable, and has a long shelf life.

Cons*:* Side effects such as headaches and migraine have been reported. It is not sold on its own to customers.

Usage*:* It is commonly used in food and pharmaceutical manufacturing such as in mouthwash and toothpaste. Ironically, it is not approved in the USA, but approved in EU in 1994 as E959.

Other Common Names*:* Neohesperidin Dihydrochalcone, NHDC

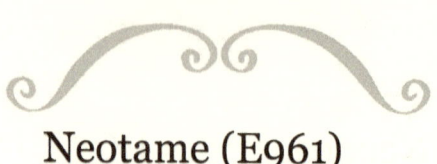

Neotame (E961)

Source and Production: Unlike other artificial sweeteners which were discovered by accident in laboratories, Neotame was born out of 20 years of trial to come up with safer forms of artificial sweetener. It contains 92% de-esterified neotame and 8% methanol. It is actually a modified and safer version of aspartame. It's manufactured by combining aspartame with 3,3-dimethylbutyraldehyde. The output is then purified, dried, and milled.

Profile: This is around 8,000 times sweeter than sugar, or 7,000 to 13,000 times depending on use. It is more heat stable compared to aspartame, making it suitable for cooking, baking, and manufacturing processed food.

Pros: It has zero calories and GI, so it's suitable for diabetics. It is also safe for people with PKU. The neotame component is excreted, while methanol (wood alcohol) is metabolized. Methanol is toxic but only a miniscule amount is present in neotame, hence it is safe. For comparison, an apple contains more methanol. It is also the cheapest sweetener (i.e. just 1% cost to achieve same sweetness of sugar).

Cons: It used mostly by food producers, not usually available to consumers. It also has negative image due to its aspartame origins.

Usage: USFDA-approved in 2002, EU-approved as E961. This is also CSPI-endorsed along with Advantame. Acceptable daily intake is 0.3mg/kg, or 44 cans of neotame-sweetened soda.

Other Common Names and Usual Brands: NutraSweet, Newtame

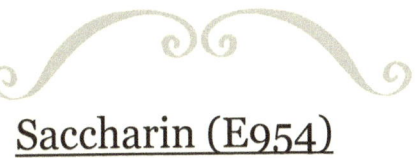

Saccharin (E954)

Source and Production: This is the first ever artificial sweetener. It was discovered by accident in 1879 by John Hopkins University chemist Constantin Fahlberg. He was working on coal tar in the lab, when he tasted a sweet substance on his hand. Saccharin is made from a synthesis of various chemicals: methyl anthranilate, nitrous acid, sulfur dioxide, chlorine, and ammonia. It started to become popular in 1960s among dieters.

Profile*:* It is 300 times sweeter than sugar, but with an unpleasant metallic or bitter taste.

Pros*:* It has zero GI and zero calories, ideal for diabetics. It is the second cheapest sweetener after Neotame. Being the oldest artificial sweetener, it is the most studied.

Cons*:* Its bad image started in 1970s when experiment rodents developed bladder cancer when fed saccharin in large amounts. It was later determined that this does not apply to humans, but the image stuck. It is not heat-stable, hence not good for cooking and baking. People on low-salt diet may need to check labels to check for sodium content as saccharin is mostly in the form of sodium salt. For those regulating sodium intake, saccharin also comes in calcium salt form.

Usage*:* It is approved all over the world. Acceptable daily intake is 15mg/kg or 56 cans of saccharin-sweetened soda.

Other Common Names*:* Pink Packets

Usual Brands*:* Sweet 'n Low, Sucron, Sweet and Low, Sweet Twin, Necta Sweet

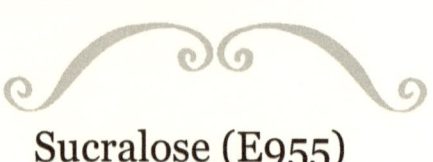

Sucralose (E955)

Source and Production: It was discovered by accident in 1976 by two researchers working with scientists from Tate & Lyle. They were experimenting on using synthetic derivatives of sucrose for industrial use, specifically as an insecticide. Leslie Hough asked Shashikant Phadnis to "test" a chlorinated sugar compound. Phadnis misheard it as "taste" so he tasted it, and found an exceptionally sweet substance. Worry not, sucralose is not an insecticide, but a chemically-modified form of table sugar made by inserting chlorine molecules into sucrose molecules. In essence, sucralose is a chlorinated derivative of sucrose.

Profile: It is 600 times sweeter than sugar. It tastes good albeit empty or flat, with little aftertaste.

Pros: With zero calories and GI, it is ideal for diabetics. It is also heat stable, making it good for cooking, baking, and manufacturing.

Cons: Specific brands add bulking agents that amp its supposedly zero caloric and glycemic content. For instance, Splenda contains Maltodextrin which has high GI per se (105). A 1-gram packet of Splenda has 3.3 calories, which is 20% of regular sugar, and 30% glycemic load of sugar. There have been reported mild side effects of sucralose such as dizziness, rashes, bloating, and cramping. While it is cheaper than table sugar, it is one of the most expensive artificial sweeteners, around twice the price of aspartame. It used to be endorsed by CSPI but not anymore as recent studies showed that it has negative impact on gut flora and may cause metabolic syndromes.

Usage: USFDA-approved in 1998, EU-approved in 2004 as E955. Acceptable daily intake is 5mg/kg or 36 cans of sucralose-sweetened soda.

Common Name: Yellow Packet

Usual Brands: Splenda, Nevella, Zerocal, Sukrana, SucraPlus, Candys, Cukren, Canderel Yellow

Summary

Artificial Sugar Substitute	Pros	Cons	Possible Side Effects
Acesulfame K (E950)	It has zero calories and carbohydrates.	Some evidence that it may cause cancer	It is widely used in mass produced products. Further research on effects is required
Advantame (E969)	It has zero calories and carbohydrates.	It is not available for consumers on its own.	Further research on effects is required
Alitame (E956)	This can be used for diabetics and those with phenylketonuria (PKU)	It is no longer produced.	
Aspartame (KE951)	Cheap to produce with zero calories and zero glycemic index	Contains phenylalanine and methanol are toxic in high doses	Reports of dizziness, headache, and blurred vision.
Aspartame-Acesulfame Salt (E962)	Has zero calories and zero glycemic index. It's also heat stable.	Similar components with aspartame	Reports of dizziness, headache, and blurred vision.
Cyclamate (E952, Sodium Cyclamate)	Cheap to produce and has zero calories and glycemic index	Old studies provided a worrying result but no human	It was tested on rats that eventually developed

		reports have been filed.	bladder tumors with long term use.
Neohesperidin DC (E959)	It is heat-stable and pH-stable, and has a long shelf life.	It masks bitter flavor and can be used in conjunction with other artificial sweeteners.	Headaches and migraine have been reported
Neotame (E961)	This can be used for diabetics and those with phenylketonuria (PKU)	Only available for manufacturers.	Since it is the same classification as aspartame, there are questions with regards to its safety.
Saccharin (E954)	One of the oldest and most studied sweetener. It has zero calories and zero glycemic index.	Saccharin comes in salt and calcium form. Read the labels prior to use to avoid potential complications	Potential allergic reaction to specific components of saccharin. Symptoms include: headache, difficulty breathing, hives and loose stools
Sucralose (E955)	Can be taken by diabetics. It can also be used for baking.	Has a flat aftertaste. It also has a negative impact on gut flora and may cause metabolic	Side effects of sucralose such as dizziness, rashes, bloating, and cramping

		syndromes.	

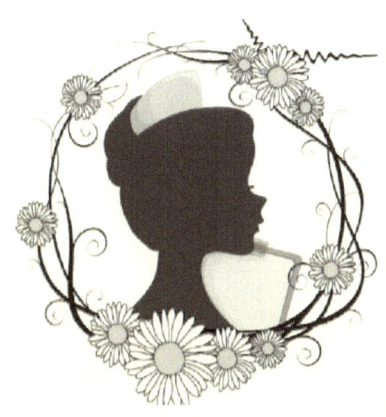

Chapter 5

Sugar Alcohols

Sugar alcohols are polyols or hybrids of sugar molecules and alcohol molecules. Despite the name, they are neither sugars nor alcohols. In fact, they do not contain alcohol or any ethanol. Food labeled as sugar-free or no sugar added usually contain sugar alcohols.

Like regular sugar, sugar alcohols are carbohydrates that occur naturally in plants, fruits, and grains, although in small quantities. Sugar alcohols usually contain just 25% calories as table sugar (4 calories per gram), are harmless to the teeth, and have low glycemic index. However, the body does not fully digest and metabolize them, and intake may result to cramping, bloating, and diarrhea. Aside from their laxative effect, they may also cause other gastric concerns for some people, especially kids.

For diabetics, these sugar types need to be accounted for when counting your daily caloric intake. Consuming large quantities of products that are labelled "sugar free" is not advised since most of these products often contain sugar alcohols.

As with other types of sugar, whether regular sugar or sugar substitutes, it is recommended to consume sugar alcohols in moderation, and as part of a well-balanced diet and healthy lifestyle.

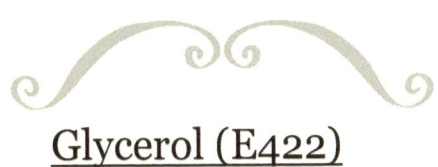

Glycerol (E422)

Source and Production: Glycerol is derived from animal or vegetable fat, sometimes from petroleum.

Profile: It is a colorless, odorless, thick, sweet, and non-toxic liquid. It has 4 calories per gram, the highest among sugar alcohols. It only has 40% sweetness compared to sugar, so it is not really used as a sweetener but for its other qualities, such as a humectant or moisture-preserving, as an antiseptic, and as a laxative. It is used more by food and medical manufacturers more than consumers.

Pros: It has low GI (3). It can be taken by diabetics but in small amounts. According to a study, it has the potential to reduce fluid loss during extensive activity when mixed with water and taken a few minutes prior to working out.

Cons: Given its low sweetness level, more grammage is needed to attain sweetness of sugar, resulting to similar levels of calories. Hence, it is not ideal for people who are trying to limit their calorie intake. Excessive intake can also cause cramping, bloating, flatulence, and diarrhea.

Usage: As a substance that prevents moisture loss, it is used as a food additive to add texture and bulk, and in sports drinks to reduce fluid loss during intense exercise, keeping athletes hydrated. It also has medical uses as an antiseptic and as treatment for burns and minor injuries. It is also a common ingredient in personal care products such as lotions, hand creams, toothpaste, and mouthwash, as well as in cough medicine. Limit dietary intake to 50 grams per day.

Other Common Names: Glycerin, Glycerine

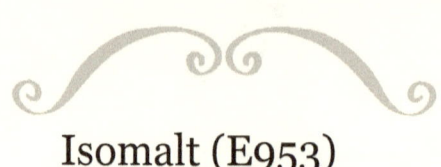

Isomalt (E953)

Source and Production: This was discovered in the 1960s as an artificial polyol synthesized from sucrose. It contains 50% glucose, 25% sorbitol, and 25% mannitol.

Profile*:* It comes in a white and odorless crystal form. It is also sold in sticks that can be melted. It has good taste with little aftertaste. It has 2.1 calories per gram, which is 53% of sugar, but it is only half as sweet as sugar.

Pros*:* Its low GI (2) makes it good for diabetics. It is a malleable and versatile baking ingredient, as well as a heat-stable and pH-stable substance suitable for cooking and manufacturing food. It does not absorb moisture, so it does not turn sticky.

Cons*:* More amount is needed to achieve the sweetness of sugar, so it is not beneficial for calorie control. It is one of the most expensive sweeteners, 5 times the price of regular sugar based on weight alone. Plus, it has a laxative effect since the body considers it fiber. It may cause discomfort or diarrhea when over-consumed.

Usage*:* It is used as coating and ingredient for sweets, hard candies, toffees, chewing gums, chocolates, and baked goods, as well as in pharmaceutical products such as supplements, cough medicine, and throat lozenges. Limit dietary intake to 20 grams per day.

Usual Brands: ClearCut Isomalt, Patisfrance Patis'Omalt

Lactitol (E966)

Source and Production: This artificial polyol was discovered in the 1920s. It is produced from lactose derived from whey, the milky byproduct of cheese.

Profile: It has good taste and texture without aftertaste. It has 2 calories per gram, which is 50% of refined sugar, but only 40% as sweet.

Pros: Its low GI (3) makes it suitable for diabetics. It dissolves easily, provides bulk, and does not absorb moisture, keeping baked goods crisp and extending shelf life. As a prebiotic, it is good to gut flora and colon health, and used to treat constipation.

Cons: Not ideal for calorie-restricted diets. It also has laxative properties, so excessive intake may lead to stomachache, gas, and diarrhea. It is expensive, about 8 times the price of regular sugar.

Usage: Common ingredient in candies, chewing gum, biscuits, chocolates, and ice cream. Limit intake to 20 grams per day.

Usual Brands: Lactitol (Danisco), Lacty (Purac Biochem)

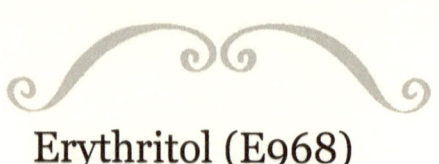

Erythritol (E968)

Source and Production: This was discovered by chemist John Stenhouse in 1848. The substance occurs naturally in some fruits and mushrooms. It is produced industrially by subjecting starch from corn to enzymatic hydrolysis to yield glucose, which is then fermented using fungus to produce erythritol. This has been used in Japan since the 1990s. It comes in crystal and powdered form, with the latter being more commonly preferred.

Profile: It has good taste with minimal aftertaste, and has mild cooling effect on the mouth. It has 0.2 calories per gram, which is 5% the calories of sugar, with 65% sweetness.

Pros: It has low GI (1) and calories, making it ideal for diabetics and weight watchers. Unlike other sugar alcohols, it is less likely to cause flatulence and irritable bowel syndrome.

Cons: Overconsumption can still lead to nausea and stomach pain or grumbling. There are also rare instances of few people being allergic to erythritol or sugar alcohols in general. It is also more expensive than regular sugar, selling for 500% to 700% more.

Usage: Used as ingredient in beverages in USA and Japan. It is also mixed with other sweeteners e.g. Truvia (with Stevia). Limit intake to 50 to 80 grams per day.

Usual Brands: C*Eridex, ZSweet, Zerose

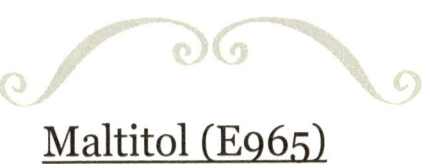

Maltitol (E965)

Source and Production*:* This occurs naturally in small amounts in chicory leaves. As a sweetener though, it is synthesized from maltose from wheat and corn. It requires a multi-step process to make: enzymatic hydrolysis, catalytic hydrogenation, and filtration.

Profile*:* It has 2.4 calories per gram, which is 60% the calories of sugar, with 90% of its sweetness.

Pros*:* It enhances subtle flavors in food especially chocolate. It also keeps food moist, while absorbing less moisture than sugar, making it handy as a coating for candies and gums.

Cons*:* This has higher GI compared to other sugar alcohols (35), and diabetics need to regulate their intake. It also has a laxative effect. This sweetener is more for manufacturers. It is average-priced.

Usage*:* Sugar-free chocolates often contain maltitol. It is also used in medicine and in moisturizers. Limit dietary intake to 50 grams per day.

Usual Brands: SweetPearl, Maltisweet

Mannitol (E421)

Source and Production: This occurs naturally in some mushrooms and algae although in small amounts. The commercially-available kind is synthesized and hydrogenated from fructose or glucose syrup.

Profile: It has good taste with minimal aftertaste, and has a cooling effect in the mouth. It has 40% calories as sugar (1.6 calories per gram) but only half as sweet.

Pros: Its low GI (2) makes is fit for diabetics. Its cooling effect makes it suitable for chewing gum. It does not absorb moisture, making it good as coating for candy and even chocolates. Useful in the medical field as a laxative, and for treating head trauma, renal failure, and cystic fibrosis. It is used to bind and coat tablets and pills. Veterinarians also use this for some treatments for dogs.

Cons: It's not really used as a sweetener and weight management sugar substitute, but more for industrial and pharmaceutical ingredient. Large doses can also be fatal, or at least have side effects such as nausea, stomach cramps, and frequent urination. Some may also be allergic to this. In addition, it is more expensive than sugar.

Usage: Limit consumption to 20 grams per day.

Usual Brands: Mannidex, Roquette

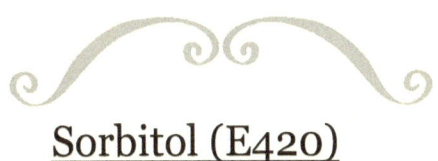

Sorbitol (E420)

Source and Production: This is a natural substance found in many fruits such as apples and pears. It is also produced by human metabolism. As a sweetener, it is synthesized from starch (corn, wheat, potato) via a multi-stage refining process of enzymatic hydrolysis and catalytic hydrogenation.

Profile: It has good taste with minimal aftertaste. It also has cooling effect in the mouth. It contains 65% calories of sugar (2.6 calories per gram), but with 55% of its sweetness.

Pros: Its low GI (4) makes it good for diabetics. It adds bulk, texture, and stiffness to sugar-free confectionery, and prolongs shelf life and regulates moisture content.

Cons: It is not suitable for calorie counters. As a laxative, it can cause diarrhea. For some people, it can cause discomfort even when ingested in small amounts. There are few who are allergic to it. On another note, dogs suffer from severe reaction when given sorbitol.

Usage: It is usually not sold on its own, although it is present in many manufactured products especially sweets and chewing gum. Limit dietary intake to 50 to 70 grams.

Xylitol (E967)

Source and Production: This is the most popular sugar alcohol. It was discovered in 1890 by German chemist Hermann Emil Fischer, and was widely used in Finland during World War 2 to cope with sugar shortage. It is natural in the sense that that humans produce it daily through metabolism, and it is present in many animals and plants. As a sweetener, it is artificially produced and refined by hydrogenating xylose then fermenting it to xylitol.

Profile: It is as sweet as sugar, but with only 62% of the calories (2.4 calories per gram). It also has a distinct mint taste that cools and refreshes the mouth.

Pros: Its low GI (12) makes it a possible option as an alternative sweetener for table sugar. It is beneficial for dental hygiene and is also used to treat middle ear infection, especially among kids.

According to a research done on the benefits of xylitol on oral health, it cannot be metabolized by plaque bacteria which in turn reduces the chances of build-up and plaque growth.

Cons: As a laxative, it can cause diarrhea when taken excessively. Considering that this sweetener isn't digested in the intestines, it can become food for gut bacteria causing gastric discomfort. There have been reports that it can increase blood glucose levels but it still requires further study.

This is very toxic for dogs: do not give xylitol to pets.

Usage: This is a common ingredient in sugar-free chewing gums, mints, candies, and oral care products like toothpaste and mouthwash. Consume as part of diet only up to 50 grams per day.

Usual Brands: Polysweet, Xylosweet, Xyla

Summary

Sugar Alcohols	Pros	Cons	Possible Side Effects
Glycerol (E422)	It can be taken by diabetics. Potentially lowers fluid loss during activity	Not as sweet as table sugar.	Excessive intake can also cause cramping, bloating, flatulence, and diarrhea.
Isomalt (E953)	It is a malleable and versatile baking ingredient, as well as a heat-stable and pH-stable substance suitable for cooking and manufacturing food.	More amount is needed to achieve the sweetness of table sugar.	It has a laxative effect since the body considers it fiber. It may cause discomfort or diarrhea when over-consumed.
Lactitol (E966)	It is a prebiotic and can extend the shelf life of baked goods.	Not for calorie restricted diets	It has laxative properties and may cause stomachache and bloating
Erythritol (E968)	It's good for diabetics and weight watchers	Overconsumption can still lead to nausea and stomach pain or grumbling	Less likely to cause flatulence and irritable bowel syndrome.
Mannitol (E421)	Useful in the medical field as a laxative, and for treating head trauma, renal failure, and cystic	Used primarily for manufacturing and industrial purposes and not as a sweetener.	Large doses can also be fatal, or at least have side effects such as nausea, stomach

	fibrosis. It is used to bind and coat tablets and pills		cramps, and frequent urination.
Sorbitol (E420)	It adds bulk, texture, and stiffness to sugar-free confectionery, and prolongs shelf life and regulates moisture content.	It shouldn't be given to dogs.	It is a laxative and can cause diarrhea.
Xylitol (E967)	As sweet as sugar and has a distinct mint taste that cools and refreshes the mouth	It isn't broken down in the intestines and may become food to gut flora causing discomfort.	It is a laxative and it can cause diarrhea when taken excessively

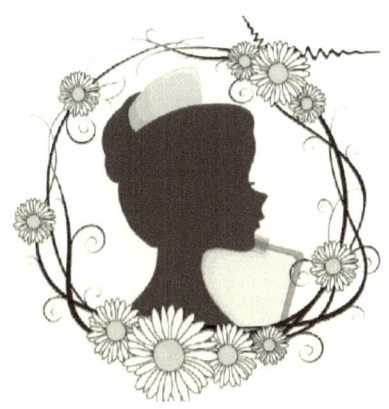

Chapter 6

Sugar Substitutes for Diabetes

After that long list of different sugar substitutes, it's easy to feel confused with the best one to use when you have diabetes or if you want to watch your glucose intake.

In the last few decades, the sugar substitutes that were used by diabetics were mostly in the form of artificial sugars such as aspartame and sucralose. However, rising health concerns have shifted the need of consumers to naturally occurring sugars.

According to a recent study in 2009, those who consume diet sodas which contain some form of artificial sweetener have higher risks of developing metabolic syndrome by 36%. Another interesting finding is that it actually raises the risk of developing type-2 diabetes by 67% when compared to those who don't consume sodas.

Newer studies have found more interesting data. In a 2014 research, it specifically studied the effects of the three common non-caloric or zero-calorie sweeteners (saccharin, sucralose and aspartame) on the metabolism and the gut flora. They tested the zero-calorie sugars on healthy mice and found that it causes "dysbiosis" and glucose intolerance on healthy mice.

There seems to be an issue with how artificial sugars are metabolized in the body. Normally, when the body detects glucose it releases insulin in order to lower the glucose levels in the blood. When using artificial sugars, the body doesn't initially react to it which causes it to stay in the body. However, these results are still inconclusive and still require further studies.

Which Sugar Substitute is Best for Diabetics?

Recently, **Stevia** has grown both in popularity and use. As a sugar substitute, it is one of the newest but also one of the most natural forms that is backed with research.

Several short-term researches were done with regards to the effect of stevia in diabetic patients. It has been widely concluded that stevia does have beneficial effects on the pancreas. Not only that but it actually increases glucose tolerance, which would highly benefit type-2 diabetics. With zero calories and zero glycemic index, it has become one of the preferable sugar substitutes to date.

When using stevia, it is best to remember that there aren't any studies regarding the long-term effects of stevia on the body. However, since it is 300 times sweeter than sugar, you only need minimal amounts to get the right sweetness. It has a long history of use in Paraguay, Brazil, Asia and Central America and has been proven safe for consumption. There haven't been any notable side effects of prolonged use but this differs on the individual and the usage. It wouldn't be wise to use this exactly like sugar since it isn't. It has different chemical properties. It's a good way of sweetening beverages and taking the sugar cravings off but use it moderately.

Lo Han Guo or **Monk Fruit** is a gourd that looks like a melon. This sweetener is grown in Southeast Asia (mostly China). This is a similar sweetener to stevia and has zero calories. It comes in extracts, powders, granules and as a dried fruit. It is over 200 times sweeter than sugar and well tolerated by the body.

There are only a few studies regarding this fruit. However, the consensus is that this sweetener does not impact blood sugar levels. There are no reports of negative side effects.

This is harder to find compared to stevia since it is expensive and difficult to produce due to its short shelf life and limited availability. There are also studies which claim that mogroside (the chemical that makes the fruit sweet) encourages the release of insulin in the pancreas, which may be bad for those who have problems with insulin sensitivity. In this condition, the pancreas is already working double time in producing insulin but it is the cells who have little or no receptors that allows the entry of glucose to be used and metabolized.

These two are the top contenders when it comes to natural sugar substitutes. However, stevia takes the top spot in terms of availability and research. Please remember to check the labels and the manufacturer before trying this out. This sweetener has already been abused by some manufacturers by including additives during processing. Check with your healthcare providers before making any changes to your diet regimen since it does impact your health and there is always a potential for allergic reactions.

MARY CONRAD

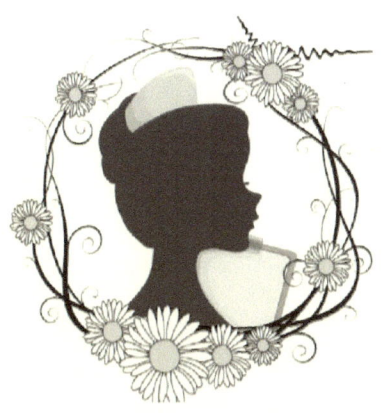

Conclusion

There are many sugar substitutes on the market. Given the wide array of choices, it can get daunting to choose a good alternative, and confusing to check the labels of packaged goods – only to find a lot of chemical-sounding sugars.

As a consumer, it is crucial to educate and familiarize yourself with these sugar jargons and terminologies so that you do not fall prey to inaccurate labels and misleading advertising. Hopefully, this book will be able to arm you with the tools necessary to be an educated consumer of sugar.

Remember: you need sweetness in your diet, but just the right level of sweetness. May you find that sweet spot with the sweetener that suits your palate and your nutritional and medical needs. Choose wisely!

Finally, if you enjoyed this book, then I'd like to ask you for a favor. Would you be kind enough to leave a review for this book on Amazon? It'd be greatly appreciated!

Follow me on Facebook (Mary Conrad) and Twitter

(@authormconrad).

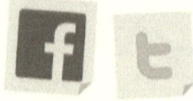

Subscribe to my newsletter to get updates on my latest book and free giveaways!
www.maryconradrn.com

If you have any suggestions or specific natural remedies that you want to have researched and written, shoot me an email at authormaryconrad@gmail.com. I'm always on the lookout for great new topics to write about. :)

Have a great day!

Thank you for taking this journey with me, and good luck!

References

Chapter 1: Overview of Regular Sugar

Sugar. (2017, April 27). Retrieved April 29, 2017, from https://en.wikipedia.org/wiki/Sugar

Sugar Addiction Facts: Cravings, Hidden Sugar, and More in Pictures. (n.d.). Retrieved April 29, 2017, from http://www.webmd.com/diet/ss/slideshow-sugar-addiction

https://www.sugar.org/wp-content/uploads/2017/02/Sugar-Science.pdf

Gunnars, K., BSc. (2016, August 18). 10 Disturbing Reasons Why Sugar is Bad For You. Retrieved April 29, 2017, from https://authoritynutrition.com/10-disturbing-reasons-why-sugar-is-bad/

Artificial sweeteners and other sugar substitutes. (2015, August 20). Retrieved April 29, 2017, from http://www.mayoclinic.org/healthy-lifestyle/nutrition-and-healthy-eating/in-depth/artificial-sweeteners/art-20046936

How Sugar is Made - the History. (n.d.). Retrieved April 30, 2017, from http://www.sucrose.com/lhist.html

Types of Sugar. (2015, June 25). Retrieved April 30, 2017, from http://www.mybakingaddiction.com/types-of-sugar/

A Complete Visual Guide to 11 Different Kinds of Sugar. (n.d.). Retrieved April 30, 2017, from http://www.thekitchn.com/a-complete-visual-guide-to-sugar-ingredient-intelligence-213715

What Are the Different Types of Sugar? (n.d.). Retrieved April 30, 2017, from https://www.sugar.org/types-of-sugar/

Daily Intake of Sugar - How Much Sugar Should You Eat Per Day? (2016, September 18). Retrieved April 30, 2017, from https://authoritynutrition.com/how-much-sugar-per-day/

Petersen, H. L. (2016, June 07). How Many Carbs Should I Eat a Day? Retrieved April 30, 2017, from http://www.healthline.com/health/lose-weight-carbs#Amount2

Carbohydrates: How carbs fit into a healthy diet. (2017, February 07). Retrieved April 30, 2017, from http://www.mayoclinic.org/healthy-lifestyle/nutrition-and-healthy-eating/in-depth/carbohydrates/art-20045705

Calories, Fat, Carbs & Protein Per Day. (n.d.). Retrieved April 30, 2017, from http://thescienceofeating.com/food-combining-how-it-works/calories-fat-carbs-protein-per-day/

Glycemic Index for Sweeteners. (n.d.). Retrieved April 30, 2017, from http://www.sugar-and-sweetener-guide.com/glycemic-index-for-sweeteners.html

Glycemic Index and Glycemic Load. (2017, January 03). Retrieved April 30, 2017, from http://lpi.oregonstate.edu/mic/food-beverages/glycemic-index-glycemic-load#table-1

Glycemic Index. (n.d.). Retrieved April 30, 2017, from http://nutritiondata.self.com/topics/glycemic-index

Types of sweetener. (n.d.). Retrieved April 30, 2017, from http://www.sugar-and-sweetener-guide.com/types-of-sweetener.html

Hilary Parker. A sweet problem: Princeton researchers find that high-fructose corn syrup prompts considerably more weight gain. Princeton University. 2010 March 22.

American Chemical Society. Soda Warning-high-fructose corn syrup linked to diabetes, new study suggests. ScienceDaily 23 Aug. 2007.

Jennifer K. Nelson R.D.,L.D. What is high-fructose corn syrup? What are the health concerns? Mayo Clinic. 2012

September 27.

Duke University Medical Center. High fructose corn syrup linked to liver scarring, research suggests. ScienceDaily. 23 Mar. 2010.

Laura G. Sánchez-Lozada, Wei Mu, Carlos Roncal, Yuri Y. Sautin, Manal Abdelmalek, Sirirat Reungjui, MyPhuong Le, Takahiko Nakagawa, Hui Y. Lan, Xuequing Yu, Richard J. Johnson. Comparison of free fructose and glucose to sucrose in the ability to cause fatty liver. European Journal of Nutrition. 2010 February. vol. 49 issue 1, pp. 1-9.

Dufault R, LeBlanc B, Schnoll R, Cornett C, Schweitzer L, Wallinga D, Hightower J, Patrick L, Lukiw WJ. Mercury from chlor-alkali plants: measured concentrations in food product sugar. Environ Health. 2009 Jan 26;8:2. doi: 10.1186/1476-069X-8-2.

Chapter 2: Modified Sugar

Agave Syrup. (n.d.). Retrieved April 30, 2017, from http://www.sugar-and-sweetener-guide.com/agave-syrup.html

Tips for Substituting Agave in Baked Goods. (n.d.). Retrieved May 01, 2017, from http://www.thekitchn.com/5-tips-on-substituting-agave-i-105651

Agave Syrup 101: Why it's a Healthy Sugar Substitute. (n.d.). Retrieved May 01, 2017, from http://kblog.lunchboxbunch.com/2009/07/agave-syrup-101-why-its-healthy-sugar.html

The difference between raw, light and amber agave nectar. (n.d.). Retrieved May 01, 2017, from http://www.wholeandnatural.com/the-difference-between-raw-light-and-amber-agave-nectar/

Barley Malt Syrup. (n.d.). Retrieved May 01, 2017, from http://www.sugar-and-sweetener-guide.com/barley-malt-syrup.html

Brown Rice Syrup. (n.d.). Retrieved May 01, 2017, from http://www.sugar-and-sweetener-guide.com/brown-rice-syrup.html

Caramel. (n.d.). Retrieved May 01, 2017, from http://www.sugar-and-sweetener-guide.com/caramel.html

Golden Syrup. (n.d.). Retrieved May 01, 2017, from http://www.sugar-and-sweetener-guide.com/golden-syrup.html

Refiners Syrup. (n.d.). Retrieved May 01, 2017, from http://www.sugar-and-sweetener-guide.com/refiners-syrup.html

High Fructose Corn Syrup. (n.d.). Retrieved May 01, 2017, from http://www.sugar-and-sweetener-guide.com/high-fructose-corn-syrup.html

Inverted Sugar. (n.d.). Retrieved May 01, 2017, from http://www.sugar-and-sweetener-guide.com/inverted-sugar.html

Chapter 3: Natural Sugar Substitutes

Natural Sweeteners. (n.d.). Retrieved May 01, 2017, from http://www.sugar-and-sweetener-guide.com/natural-sweeteners.html

8 Healthy Sweeteners to Use Instead of Sugar. (2017, April 27). Retrieved May 01, 2017, from https://authoritynutrition.com/natural-sugar-substitutes/

Stevia and Sugar Substitutes. (n.d.). Retrieved May 01, 2017, from http://www.webmd.com/diet/stevia-sugar-substitutes#1

Mailonline, M. M. (2015, August 11). Molasses, coconut palm and monk fruit: The 10 best natural substitutes for sugar... and which ones have the LEAST calories. Retrieved May 01, 2017, from http://www.dailymail.co.uk/femail/food/article-3191361/The-10-best-natural-substitutes-refined-sugar.html

Glick | 2 COMMENTS, L. (n.d.). It's Official: Sugar is the New Crack. Retrieved May 01, 2017, from http://www.totalbeauty.com/content/slideshows/natural-sugar-alternatives/page1

Monk Fruit In The Raw. (n.d.). Retrieved May 01, 2017, from http://www.intheraw.com/products/monk-fruit-in-the-raw

Greenfield, B. (2014, August 08). 10 Natural Alternatives to Sugar: How Healthy Are They Really? Retrieved May 01, 2017, from https://www.yahoo.com/beauty/10-natural-alternatives-to-sugar-how-healthy-are-they-93420596832.html

Gartland, A. (n.d.). Naturally Sweet: 4 Chemical-Free Sugar Substitutes. Retrieved May 01, 2017, from http://www.oprah.com/health/sugar-substitutes-healthy-natural-sweeteners

Genta, S., Cabrera, W., Habib, N., Pons, J., Carillo, I. M., Grau, A., & Sánchez, S. (2009). Yacon syrup: beneficial effects on obesity and insulin resistance in humans. *Clinical Nutrition*, *28*(2), 182-187.

https://www.ncbi.nlm.nih.gov/pubmed/19254816

Cane Juice. (n.d.). Retrieved May 01, 2017, from http://www.sugar-and-sweetener-guide.com/canejuice.html

Coconut Palm Sugar. (n.d.). Retrieved May 01, 2017, from http://www.sugar-and-sweetener-guide.com/coconut-palm-sugar.html

Benfit, E. (2016, July 07). How to Make Your Own Date Sugar. Retrieved May 01, 2017, from http://butterbeliever.com/how-to-make-your-own-date-sugar/

Shreeves, R. (2014, November 10). Are dates the new low glycemic sugar substitute? Retrieved May 01, 2017, from https://www.fromthegrapevine.com/israeli-kitchen/are-dates-new-low-glycemic-sugar-substitute#!

The Sweet Subtlety of Date Sugar. (n.d.). Retrieved May 02, 2017, from http://www.thekitchn.com/ingredient-spotlight-date-sugar-176751

Lucuma Fruit Powder, Benefits as an Alternative Sweetener. (n.d.). Retrieved May 02, 2017, from http://www.superfoods-for-superhealth.com/lucuma.html

Kemeny, M. (2015, January 28). 3 Reasons Lucuma Powder is the Superfood to Lower Your Sugar Intake (And Lose Weight!). Retrieved May 02, 2017, from http://maureenkemeny.com/use-superfood-lower-sugar-intake-lose-weight/

Maple Syrup. (n.d.). Retrieved May 02, 2017, from http://www.sugar-and-sweetener-guide.com/maple-syrup.html

E. (n.d.). Maple and Pancake Syrup Taste Test. Retrieved May 02, 2017, from http://www.epicurious.com/archive/everydaycooking/tastetests/maple-syrup-taste-test

Bowe, T. (2017, April 11). The 5 Best Maple Syrups. Retrieved May 02, 2017, from https://gearpatrol.com/2015/03/27/best-maple-syrup/

Molasses. (n.d.). Retrieved May 02, 2017, from http://www.sugar-and-sweetener-guide.com/molasses.html

Nutritional Comparisons of Blackstrap Molasses Brands. (n.d.). Retrieved May 02, 2017, from https://www.earthclinic.com/remedies/molasses-brand-comparisons.html

Sorghum Syrup. (n.d.). Retrieved May 02, 2017, from http://www.sugar-and-sweetener-guide.com/sorghum-syrup.html

Glycyrrhizin. (n.d.). Retrieved May 02, 2017, from http://www.sugar-and-sweetener-guide.com/glycyrrhizin.html

Luo Han Guo (also known as Monk Fruit). (n.d.). Retrieved May 02, 2017, from http://www.sugar-and-sweetener-guide.com/luo-han-guo.html

Grier, A. J. (n.d.). Finally, sampling miracle fruit tablets. Retrieved May 02, 2017, from http://www.jacobgrier.com/blog/archives/1220.html

Cox, D. (2014, May 29). The 'Miracle' Berry That Could Replace Sugar. Retrieved May 02, 2017, from https://www.theatlantic.com/health/archive/2014/05/can-miraculin-solve-the-global-obesity-epidemic/371657/

Miraculin. (2017, April 04). Retrieved May 02, 2017, from https://en.wikipedia.org/wiki/Miraculin

Fowler, A. (2008, April 28). The miracle berry. Retrieved May 02, 2017, from http://news.bbc.co.uk/2/hi/uk_news/magazine/7367548.stm

Stevia. (n.d.). Retrieved May 02, 2017, from http://www.sugar-and-sweetener-guide.com/stevia.html

The Five Best-Tasting No-Cal Stevia Sweeteners. (2015, June 07). Retrieved May 02, 2017, from http://www.prevention.com/eatclean/stevia-brand-taste-test

FAQ. (n.d.). Retrieved May 02, 2017, from https://www.stevia.com/faq/

Chapter 4: Artificial Sugar Substitutes

Myers, W. (2015, September 13). Complete List of Artificial Sweeteners. Retrieved May 02, 2017, from https://liveto110.com/complete-list-of-artificial-sweeteners/

Saulo, A. A. (2005). Sugars and sweeteners in foods.

https://www.ctahr.hawaii.edu/oc/freepubs/pdf/FST-16.pdf

Sugar Substitutes. (2015, May 15). Retrieved May 02, 2017, from http://midtownnutrition.net/2015/05/15/sugar-substitutes/

Acesulfame K. (n.d.). Retrieved May 02, 2017, from http://www.sugar-and-sweetener-guide.com/acesulfameK.html

Karstadt, M. L. (2006). Testing needed for acesulfame potassium, an artificial sweetener. Environmental health perspectives, 114(9), A516.

https://www.ncbi.nlm.nih.gov/pmc/articles/PMC1570055/pdf/ehp0114-a0516a.pdf

Acesulfame potassium. (2017, April 18). Retrieved May 02, 2017, from https://en.wikipedia.org/wiki/Acesulfame_potassium

Acesulfame-K Toxicity Information Center. (n.d.). Retrieved May 02, 2017, from http://www.holisticmed.com/acek/

Stop the Filthy Food Act. (n.d.). Retrieved May 03, 2017, from https://cspinet.org/eating-healthy/chemical-cuisine

Everything You Need to Know About Acesulfame Potassium - Nutrition Express Articles. (n.d.). Retrieved May 03, 2017, from https://www.nutritionexpress.com/article   index/vitamins supplements a-z/showarticle.aspx?id=120

DrSwati Verma . (2015, March 01). Sugar substitutes . Retrieved May   03,   2017,   from https://www.slideshare.net/drswativerma2/sugar-substitutes-ppt

What is Acesulfame Potassium, and is it Good or Bad For You? (2016,   August   17).   Retrieved   May   03,   2017,   from https://authoritynutrition.com/acesulfame-potassium-good-or-bad/

Franz, M., MS, RD, LD. (n.d.). AMOUNTS OF SWEETENERS IN POPULAR DIET SODAS. Retrieved May 4, 2017, from http://static.diabetesselfmanagement.com/pdfs/DSM0310_012.pdf

Advantame. (n.d.). Retrieved May 03, 2017, from http://www.sugar-and-sweetener-guide.com/advantame.html

Advantame. (2017, May 03). Retrieved May 03, 2017, from https://en.wikipedia.org/wiki/Advantame

FDA Approves New No-Calorie Sweetener. (n.d.). Retrieved May 03, 2017, from http://www.medscape.com/viewarticle/825427

Alitame. (n.d.). Retrieved May 04, 2017, from http://www.sugar-and-sweetener-guide.com/alitame.html

Ehrenberg, R. (2015, December 30). Artificial sweeteners may tip scales toward metabolic problems. Retrieved May 04, 2017, from https://www.sciencenews.org/article/artificial-sweeteners-may-tip-scales-toward-metabolic-problems

Alitame. (2017, April 18). Retrieved May 04, 2017, from https://en.wikipedia.org/wiki/Alitame

Hills, S. (2008, June 22). Sweetener production stopped due to high costs. Retrieved May 04, 2017, from http://www.foodnavigator-usa.com/Suppliers2/Sweetener-production-stopped-due-to-high-costs

Aspartame. (n.d.). Retrieved May 04, 2017, from http://www.sugar-and-sweetener-guide.com/aspartame.html

Aspartame is, By Far, The Most Dangerous Substance on The Market That is Added to Foods. (n.d.). Retrieved May 04, 2017, from http://aspartame.mercola.com/

Aspartame-Acesulfame Salt. (n.d.). Retrieved May 04, 2017, from http://www.sugar-and-sweetener-guide.com/aspartame-acesulfame-salt.html

Aspartame-acesulfame salt. (2017, April 18). Retrieved May 04, 2017, from https://en.wikipedia.org/wiki/Aspartame-acesulfame_salt

Cyclamate. (n.d.). Retrieved May 04, 2017, from http://www.sugar-and-sweetener-guide.com/cyclamate.html

Takayama, S., Renwick, A. G., Johansson, S. L., Thorgeirsson, U. P., Tsutsumi, M., Dalgard, D. W., & Sieber, S. M. (2000). Long-term toxicity and carcinogenicity study of cyclamate in nonhuman primates. Toxicological Sciences, 53(1), 33-39.

Sodium cyclamate. (2017, April 18). Retrieved May 04, 2017, from https://en.wikipedia.org/wiki/Sodium_cyclamate

Kaufman, L. (1999, August 20). Michael Sveda, the Inventor Of Cyclamates, Dies at 87. Retrieved May 04, 2017, from http://www.nytimes.com/1999/08/21/business/michael-sveda-the-inventor-of-cyclamates-dies-at-87.html

Neohesperidin DC. (n.d.). Retrieved May 04, 2017, from http://www.sugar-and-sweetener-guide.com/Neohesperidin-DC.html

Neohesperidin dihydrochalcone. (2017, April 18). Retrieved May 04, 2017, from https://en.wikipedia.org/wiki/Neohesperidin_dihydrochalcone

Neotame. (n.d.). Retrieved May 04, 2017, from http://www.sugar-and-sweetener-guide.com/neotame.html

Neotame. (n.d.). Retrieved May 04, 2017, from http://www.neotame.com/

Neotame. (n.d.). Retrieved May 05, 2017, from https://pubchem.ncbi.nlm.nih.gov/compound/Neotame#section=Mechanism-of-Action

Center for Food Safety and Applied Nutrition. (n.d.). Food Additives & Ingredients - Additional Information about High-Intensity Sweeteners Permitted for use in Food in the United States. Retrieved May 05, 2017, from

https://www.fda.gov/food/ingredientspackaginglabeling/foodadd
itivesingredients/ucm397725.htm

Neotame. (2017, April 18). Retrieved May 05, 2017, from
https://en.wikipedia.org/wiki/Neotame

Preidt, R. (2014, May 20). FDA approves new artificial sweetener.
Retrieved May 05, 2017, from
http://www.cbsnews.com/news/fda-approves-new-artificial-
sweetener/

MA, J., & CHEN, M. (n.d.). Neotame – A Powerful and Safe
Sweetener. Retrieved May 05, 2017, from
http://www.cfs.gov.hk/english/multimedia/multimedia_pub/mul
timedia_pub_fsf_45_02.html

Saccharin. (n.d.). Retrieved May 05, 2017, from
http://www.sugar-and-sweetener-guide.com/saccharin.html

Artificial Sweeteners and Cancer. (n.d.). Retrieved May 05, 2017,
from https://www.cancer.gov/about-cancer/causes-
prevention/risk/diet/artificial-sweeteners-fact-sheet

Saccharin. (2017, April 18). Retrieved May 05, 2017, from
https://en.wikipedia.org/wiki/Saccharin

Sucralose. (n.d.). Retrieved May 05, 2017, from http://www.sugar-and-sweetener-guide.com/sucralose.html

CSPI Downgrades Splenda From "Safe" to "Caution". (n.d.). Retrieved May 05, 2017, from https://cspinet.org/new/201306121.html

Weizmann Institute of Science. (n.d.). Certain gut bacteria may induce metabolic changes following exposure to artificial sweeteners. Retrieved May 05, 2017, from https://www.sciencedaily.com/releases/2014/09/140917131634.htm

Sucralose. (2017, May 04). Retrieved May 05, 2017, from https://en.wikipedia.org/wiki/Sucralosehttps://www.ncbi.nlm.nih.gov/pubmed/25842566

Tandel, K. R. (2011). Sugar substitutes: Health controversy over perceived benefits. Journal of Pharmacology and Pharmacotherapeutics, 2(4), 236. https://www.ncbi.nlm.nih.gov/pmc/articles/PMC3198517/

Weihrauch, M. R., & Diehl, V. (2004). Artificial sweeteners—do they bear a carcinogenic risk? Annals of Oncology, 15(10), 1460-1465. https://www.ncbi.nlm.nih.gov/pubmed/15367404

Karstadt, M. (2010). Inadequate toxicity tests of food additive acesulfame. International journal of occupational and environmental health, 16(1), 89-96.

https://www.ncbi.nlm.nih.gov/pubmed/20166324

Chapter 5: Sugar Alcohols

Joslin Diabetes Center. (n.d.). What Are Sugar Alcohols? Retrieved May 05, 2017, from http://www.joslin.org/info/what_are_sugar_alcohols.html

Sugar alcohol. (2017, April 29). Retrieved May 05, 2017, from https://en.wikipedia.org/wiki/Sugar_alcohol

Sugar Alcohols: Good or Bad? (2016, August 18). Retrieved May 05, 2017, from https://authoritynutrition.com/sugar-alcohols-good-or-bad/

Sugar Alcohols. (n.d.). Retrieved May 05, 2017, from http://www.diabetes.org/food-and-fitness/food/what-can-i-eat/understanding-carbohydrates/sugar-alcohols.html

Glycerol. (n.d.). Retrieved May 05, 2017, from http://www.sugar-and-sweetener-guide.com/glycerol.html

GLYCEROL: Uses, Side Effects, Interactions and Warnings. (n.d.). Retrieved May 05, 2017, from http://www.webmd.com/vitamins-supplements/ingredientmono-4-

glycerol.aspx?activeingredientid=4

Glycerol. (2017, May 02). Retrieved May 05, 2017, from https://en.wikipedia.org/wiki/Glycerol

Isomalt. (n.d.). Retrieved May 05, 2017, from http://www.sugar-and-sweetener-guide.com/isomalt.html

Isomalt. (2017, April 18). Retrieved May 06, 2017, from https://en.wikipedia.org/wiki/Isomalt

Isomalt Sugar - Pure Isomalt for Chefs & Sugar Artists. (n.d.). Retrieved May 06, 2017, from http://www.makeyourownmolds.com/isomalt

Isomalt. (2015, October 22). Retrieved May 06, 2017, from http://caloriecontrol.org/isomalt/

Lactitol. (n.d.). Retrieved May 06, 2017, from http://www.sugar-and-sweetener-guide.com/lactitol.html

Lactitol. (2017, April 18). Retrieved May 06, 2017, from https://en.wikipedia.org/wiki/Lactitol

Maydeo, A. (2010). Lactitol or lactulose in the treatment of chronic constipation: result of a systematic. https://www.ncbi.nlm.nih.gov/pubmed/21510584

Erythritol. (n.d.). Retrieved May 06, 2017, from http://www.sugar-and-sweetener-guide.com/erythritol.html

RD, J. R. (2016, March 21). The Benefits and Risks of Erythritol as a Sweetener. Retrieved May 06, 2017, from http://www.livestrong.com/article/556918-the-disadvantages-of-erythritol/

Maltitol. (n.d.). Retrieved May 06, 2017, from http://www.sugar-and-sweetener-guide.com/maltitol.html

Mannitol. (n.d.). Retrieved May 06, 2017, from http://www.sugar-and-sweetener-guide.com/mannitol.html

Sorbitol. (n.d.). Retrieved May 06, 2017, from http://www.sugar-and-sweetener-guide.com/sorbitol.html

Xylitol. (n.d.). Retrieved May 06, 2017, from http://www.sugar-and-sweetener-guide.com/xylitol.html

Söderling, E. (2009). Controversies around xylitol. European journal of dentistry, 3(2), 81. https://www.ncbi.nlm.nih.gov/pmc/articles/PMC2676064/

Xylitol. (2017, May 06). Retrieved May 07, 2017, from https://en.wikipedia.org/wiki/Xylitol

Wingo, J. E., Casa, D. J., Berger, E. M., Dellis, W. O., Knight, J. C., & McClung, J. M. (2004). Influence of a pre-exercise glycerol hydration beverage on performance and physiologic function during mountain-bike races in the heat. Journal of athletic training, 39(2), 169. https://www.ncbi.nlm.nih.gov/pmc/articles/PMC419512/

Chapter 6

Nettleton, J. A., Lutsey, P. L., Wang, Y., Lima, J. A., Michos, E. D., & Jacobs, D. R. (2009, April 01). Diet Soda Intake and Risk of Incident Metabolic Syndrome and Type 2 Diabetes in the Multi-Ethnic Study of Atherosclerosis (MESA). Retrieved May 07, 2017, from http://care.diabetesjournals.org/content/32/4/688.full?wptouch_preview_theme=enabled

Suez, J., Korem, T., Zeevi, D., Zilberman-Schapira, G., Thaiss, C. A., Maza, O., Elinav, E. (2014, September 17). Artificial sweeteners induce glucose intolerance by altering the gut microbiota. Retrieved May 07, 2017, from http://www.nature.com/nature/journal/v514/n7521/abs/nature1 3793.html

Assaei, R., Mokarram, P., Dastghaib, S., Darbandi, S., Darbandi, M., Zal, F., ... & Omrani, G. H. R. (2016). Hypoglycemic Effect of Aquatic Extract of Stevia in Pancreas of Diabetic Rats: PPARγ-dependent Regulation or Antioxidant Potential. Avicenna journal of medical biotechnology, 8(2), 65. https://www.ncbi.nlm.nih.gov/pubmed/27141265

Goyal, S.K., Samsher and Goyal, R.K. (2010). Stevia (Stevia rebaudiana) a bio-sweetener: A review. *International Journal of Food Sciences and Nutrition,* 61, 1, 1-10.Kobylewski, S. and Eckhert, C.D. (2008). Toxicology of rabaudioside A: A review. Retrieved April 18, 2017.

Author Biography

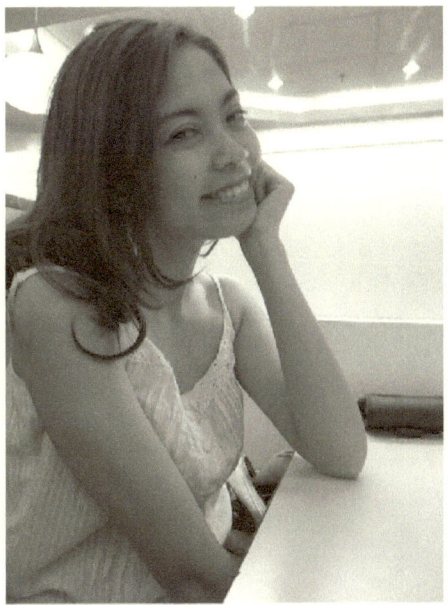

Mary Conrad is a Registered Nurse, who has a strong interest in natural remedies. As a mother, she believes in a holistic approach to health and well-being. Even though she graduated in the health profession, which usually advocates pharmaceutical medication, she believes that prevention is the best step towards health. Backed with scientific research, she wrote these books for both personal information and for others who share the same passion for holistic wellness. It's all about knowing the best natural ways to prevent disease and remedy current health problems. Like every health care provider, she believes in doing no harm, and promoting health. Take a step towards health, and towards nature.

CHECK OUT MY OTHER BOOKS:

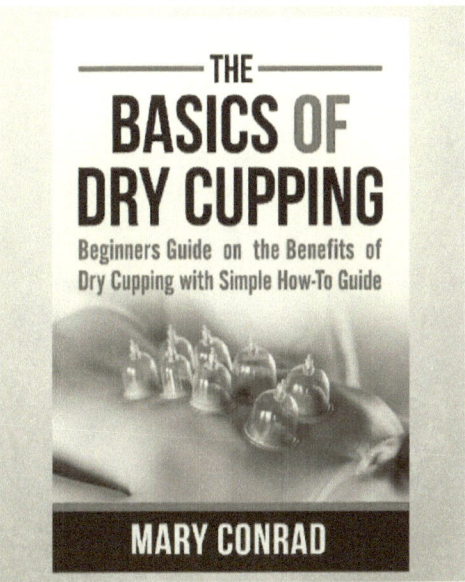

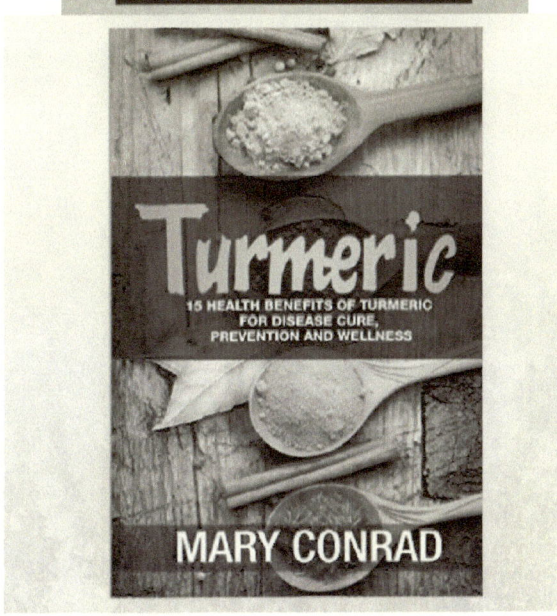

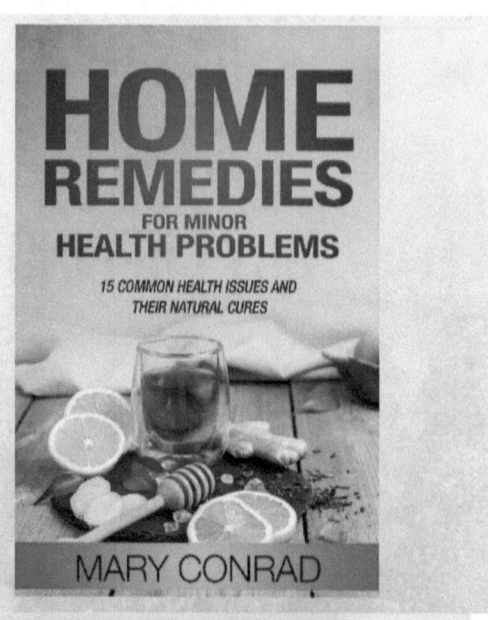

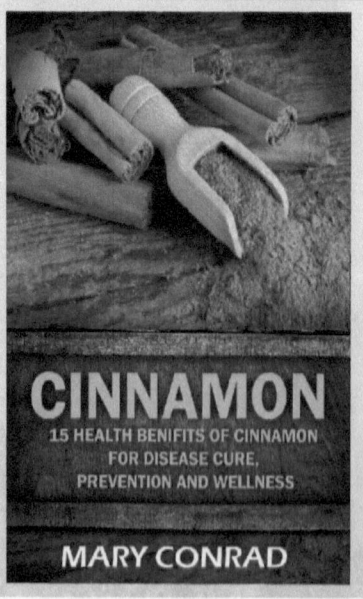

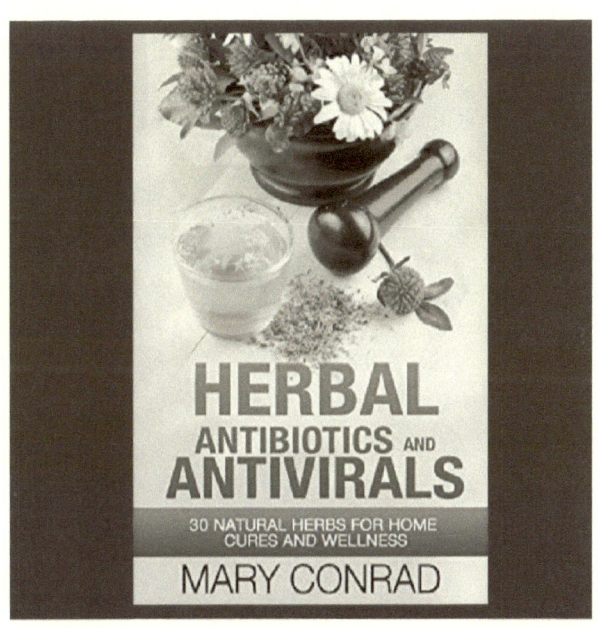

www.ingramcontent.com/pod-product-compliance
Lightning Source LLC
Chambersburg PA
CBHW020536290526
45786CB00002B/913